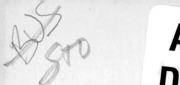
Nick Siano['s ...] managing, and living with HIV infection is a [book] I had dreamed someone would write. It is complete, up-to-date, direct, and practical, but most importantly it tells the truth. I will recommend it to all my patients and I know that having this book as their companion will become a very important part of their treatment.

—DEEPAK CHOPRA, M.D., author of
Quantum Healing, Perfect Health,
and *Unconditional Life*

Nick Siano's *No Time to Wait* explains the treatment options for people living with HIV in concise, methodical, easy to understand terms. He begins with explaining how to develop a good relationship with your physician and/or medical team and provides a complete resource. Nick's positive attitude is pervasive throughout the book. He writes in a human tone, helping us to do what we can at our own pace.

—JANET GOLDBERG, program director,
South Bronx Neighborhood AIDS Project

Nicky's book *No Time to Wait* is the most encompassing, compassionate, up-to-date, spiritual, and positive work I have ever read on HIV. It will help to break the chains that surround the concept of HIV+. "If the *only* people who had AIDS were rich ones, we would have a cure" is a statement that Nicky's book will help to change.

—JOHN S. LICHTENSTEIN, M.D., Family Practice,
Acupuncture, Alcoholism and Chemical
Dependence, and president of the
medical staff, Ellenville Hospital

Nick Siano's *No Time to Wait* is an impressively thorough state-of-the-art compendium that does exactly what it says it does, which is to provide a guide to treating, managing, and living with HIV infection. The ever-growing mushrooming of information and advice all too often has the effect of creating confusion and anxiety, which only adds to feelings of helplessness and despair in the person with HIV infection. The clarity and organization of Nick Siano's book is a godsend and its timeliness is aptly conveyed by his title, *No Time to Wait.*

—GANGA STONE, executive director,
God's Love We Deliver

A Message to HIV+ Patients

and Caregivers

Evidence that we are gaining ground against HIV infection is all around us. People are surviving and maintaining good health far longer than the media would have us believe. Every month scores of medical publications describe research, treatment, and combined strategies for caring for HIV-infected people. But only a tiny percentage of this information reaches the lay public, and only the most conventional treatments reach the practicing medical community.

No Time to Wait is a positive, practical approach to solving the problems, both medical and emotional, experienced by people with HIV. It has been designed to bring the full range of treatment information to HIV+ patients and their medical caregivers, explain the disease and its symptoms in terms everyone can clearly understand, provide information on controlling the spread of the virus, and give access to a wide range of drug and alternative therapy options. Its goal is to give people with HIV the tools they need to participate fully in their own treatment. HIV is now a disease people can live with—not die from. It is the mission of *No Time to Wait* to tell you how.

NO TIME
TO WAIT

A COMPLETE GUIDE TO TREATING, MANAGING, AND LIVING WITH HIV INFECTION

Nick Siano

with Suzanne Lipsett

BANTAM BOOKS

NEW YORK · TORONTO · LONDON · SYDNEY · AUCKLAND

This book is dedicated to Eileen Pagan for getting me started, and to Tim Kelley for helping me finish

This book is not intended as a substitute for the medical advice of physicians. The reader should regularly consult a physician in matters relating to his or her health and particularly in respect to any symptoms which may require diagnosis or medical attention. As no one course of treatment is right for everyone, readers should also speak with their own doctor or doctors about their individual needs before embarking on a course of treatment and/or if any change in treatment is desired.

NO TIME TO WAIT
A Bantam Book / June 1993

Grateful acknowledgment is made for permission to reprint the following:

From "Management of HIV Disease: One Physician's Approach," by Dr. Bernard Bihari, in *BETA*, November 1991. Reprinted by permission of the author.

Adaptation of "Nutrition and HIV," by D. Rakower, in *Bellevue Hospital Center AIDS Patient Handbook,* J. Kalinoski, ed. (New York: New York City Health and Hospital Corporation, 1991). Reprinted by permission of the author.

Excerpt from *Surviving AIDS,* by Michael Callen. Copyright © 1990 by Michael Callen. Reprinted by permission of HarperCollins Publishers, Inc.

Illustration of the HIV virus in cross section, by George V. Kelvin, originally published in *Scientific American,* October 1988. Reprinted by permission of the illustrator.

Illustration of viral reproduction, by Hank Iken, originally published in *Scientific American,* October 1988. Reprinted by permission of *Scientific American.*

Library of Congress Cataloging-in-Publication Data

Siano, Nick
    No time to wait : a complete guide to treating, managing, and living with HIV infection / Nick Siano with Suzanne Lipsett.
        p.   cm.
    Includes bibliographical references and index.
    ISBN 0-553-37176-2 : $12.95
    1. HIV infections—Popular works.   I. Lipsett, Suzanne.
II. Title.
RC607.A26S497   1993
616.97'92—dc20
                                                                    93-16398
                                                                    CIP

Published simultaneously in the United States and Canada

Bantam Books are published by Bantam Books, a division of Bantam Doubleday Dell Publishing Group, Inc. Its trademark, consisting of the words "Bantam Books" and the portrayal of a rooster, is Registered in U.S. Patent and Trademark Office and in other countries. Marca Registrada. Bantam Books, 1540 Broadway, New York, New York 10036.

PRINTED IN THE UNITED STATES OF AMERICA

FFG   0   9   8   7   6   5   4   3   2   1

Contents

PART III: LIVING WITH HIV INFECTION

Foreword

Nick Siano's book is an important contribution to the growing reality that HIV infection is in the process of becoming a manageable, treatable, preventable, and ultimately curable illness. My hope is that *No Time to Wait*, which provides much intelligent and sensitive guidance and information, will itself be a catalyst for the individual and for the social changes required to further accelerate the healing of AIDS.

As a physician who currently cares for many HIV-infected individuals in New York City, I am currently participating, along with other physicians, in the rapid growth of scientific knowledge and clinical expertise that is enabling our patients to live longer and better. I believe it is possible for many of our patients to survive HIV disease. As physicians we must regularly make the best use of available knowledge and individualize treatments to increase the chances of our patients living long enough to receive more effective future treatments that are on the way.

The notion that AIDS is an incurable disease, in addition to being untrue, serves to justify a lack of commitment and vision that itself inhibits progress. AIDS is ultimately curable and it is urgent that we respond individually, socially, spiritually, politically, and emotionally to this potential. The quicker the response the more lives that will be saved.

In my medical practice I have been privileged to meet a most extraordinary group of people living with HIV disease. These individuals have a passion for life, a graciousness and generosity of spirit, and an extraordinary courage. To live with the uncertainty, the physical and emotional stress that a diagnosis of HIV brings requires strength and love. My patients have shown me that they are not victims, but rather heroes fighting for their lives and, as I will explain later, fighting for our collective survival. It is an extraordinary privilege to witness the courage, intelligence, and humor of my patients as they struggle physically, intellectually, emotionally, and spiritually to live with HIV.

Nick's book communicates more than just a truckload of valuable information. Nick intuitively understands that the healing process itself depends upon a kind of openness and caringness which allows for dialogue between doctor and patient, patient and illness, scientist and nature, in which any and all kinds of questions are permitted and encouraged. Unfortunately, these values have often been lost in the current practice of medical and scientific research, in which truth is just one of a number of considerations that guide current standards of practice and research.

People living with HIV consider everything from the latest experimental drugs developed by pharmaceutical companies, to herbal treatments, nutritional approaches, psychotherapy, and healing processes such as acupuncture, body work, and visualization, as part of their treatment program. Nick respects these interests and supplies information about a whole range of approaches. The art of medicine involves selecting and integrating the approaches that best foster the health of the individual patient. Together the doctor and patient must be willing to learn, be flexible, and readjust the therapies based on the individual's response to treatment. And sometimes doctor and patient must be willing to move into the unknown, where there is no sure guide in certain situations. Indeed, some of my patients are surviving with problems for which, at the time of diagnosis, there were no clearcut treatments; and yet, through respectful and rational clinical experimentation, successful treatments were found. And some of my patients have gone beyond my own knowledge and skills and found treatments and ways of surviving with problems I could not help them with.

Healing AIDS, and healing in general, is a comprehensive learning process that is multidimensional. I believe that the same tools and awarenesses we need to acquire to heal AIDS at an individual and global level are necessary for us to survive collectively on this planet. I would like to dedicate this foreword to all of the individuals living with HIV, who have taught us all so very much.

—PAUL CURTIS BELLMAN, M.D.

Introduction

My motivation for writing this book has been to offer options and to spread the word that there are people living with HIV infection. My best friend died of AIDS in 1983, and I knew that if I did not become part of the solution, I would be left feeling the fear, helplessness, and hopelessness that anyone experiencing or touched by HIV knows too well. I preferred to run into action and avoid those feelings at all costs.

I searched for an answer, and now I work as an HIV specialist in New York City, disseminating treatment information to clients and working closely with doctors who prescribe treatment interventions I recommend. Now I've put together *No Time to Wait: A Complete Guide to Treating, Managing, and Living with HIV Infection.* I've drawn on extensive up-to-the-minute research and my experiences as a professional in the field; I've also tried to offer you the emotional support that goes hand in hand with the successful management of any chronic illness.

Recently, during a consultation, the mother of a client asked me why I know more about HIV infection than most doctors. The answer is no mystery. Since my job requires that I read constantly to update my knowledge of HIV treatment options, I have more time to research new therapies than doctors do. It is simply a matter of first reading and collecting information and then following the cases of patients on various therapies. I currently read seventeen HIV-specific publications, cover to cover, every month; it has been my job for the last six years. In addition, many doctors did not go to school during the age of AIDS; I did. Twenty-five percent of my undergraduate courses were HIV specific.

I do not in any way disregard the hard work and long hours that doctors have contributed toward HIV and AIDS patient care, but I do know that in this pandemic, if doctors do not have enough time to read extensively and contact colleagues to discuss new therapies, they will have a great deal of difficulty staying on top of the daily changes in treatment options for HIV infection.

I have gathered information from over a thousand sources for this book and have tried to present this information in an uncensored fashion so that you can make up your own mind and participate fully in your own treatment, instead of leaving all your decisions to a health-care provider. Added to my research is the fact that I have done over a thousand consultations with HIV+ individuals, during which I helped people learn to interpret their bloodwork and design an appropriate treatment program, combining different approaches for maximum benefit and monitoring the results. Everyone thinks his or her way is best, but I believe all treatment methods have their benefits, and a combination of the best options—depending upon the individual needs and goals of an HIV+ person—can offer additional advantages and possible gain. For instance, an acupuncture program combined with a regimen of AZT, a combination I have recommended for years, made news at the 1992 International AIDS Conference in Amsterdam as a beneficial, complementary method of treatment. One study presented at the conference cited acupuncture as "extending survival and substantially reducing side effects from HIV-related drugs."

Toward the end of this book, in Chapters 19 (Keeping Current) and 20 (A Resource Guide), you will find all the tools that I have used to stay abreast of treatment information. You, too, can read and learn ... and maybe write the next book on HIV treatment options. In the meantime, keep your doctor informed and you might benefit with more options and a longer life.

This book was meant to open your eyes, support you while doing so, and wish you well on your journey. For if you are HIV+ or working with people who are, you are on a journey where you might meet your true self and experience feelings that are sad, happy, frightening, maddening, and very real. You might also experience the healing power of love.

Physical healing is a wonderful and joyous thing, and emotional healing is a spiritual high. Although this book is a book about hope and life, many of us will "heal" into death, and this is a possibility that should be faced. Be not afraid, since fear will only taint your decisions. Instead, explore and seek answers.

You deserve the truth.

Notes from the Author

This book has been reviewed in detail for accuracy by a panel of medical experts on HIV infection and was current when it went to press (March 1993). However, the book is designed and intended as an information resource, not a prescription for treatment. Its purpose is to arm you with the latest data so you can participate fully in your medical treatment and make informed decisions. Before acting on information you find here, verify it with your health-care providers and/or the appropriate agency. Do not mistake responsible, informed self-care for casual, unverified self-treatment.

In the summer of 1992, I attended the Eighth International AIDS Conference in Amsterdam. The information in that conference was disseminated in large books containing small descriptions, called abstracts, of research studies. Throughout this book, whenever I refer to information from the conference, I cite the number of the abstract in parentheses; for example: (PoB 3362). This means that if you have access to the conference reports, you can easily look up the research and read the documentation yourself.

The term *toxicity* arises often in this book. The way I define the term, toxicity is an unwanted effect from a substance that is to some degree harmful. Where drugs are concerned, toxicity can range from mild to extremely hazardous.

All the substances described here as toxic can also be beneficial. In addition, if a treatment is toxic for one patient, it may not be for another. To decide whether or not to take a treatment with toxic side effects, you will need to carefully discuss with your physician both the benefits and the risks and then make a personal decision as to whether the benefits outweigh the risks. One of my objectives in the book is to equip you with the information you need to make this assessment.

PART I

FUNDAMENTALS

CHAPTER 1

Hiring a Physician

First things first. This book is not going to feed into the negative, fatalistic messages circling all around us. You've already heard enough of those. It's a difficult diagnosis to hear, but *finding out you are HIV+ is not the end of the world*—and you don't have to listen to anyone who thinks it is.

This book has one underlying message: *You can live with HIV.* Like many people right now going about their lives symptom-free or managing their symptoms as they arise, you can manage HIV infection. To do that you need a strong support network, up-to-date information, and a medical team you can trust. Finding the right medical people is no small task—it can determine the course your treatment takes.

However, upon diagnosis, one thing takes precedence above all else: ensuring that you are not alone. Your health depends on your emotional well-being, and that in turn depends on your sense of connection to the world. Before doing anything else, find, build, and tap in to a support network of people who

- aren't inclined to pamper you
- don't gaze at you sadly, immobilized
- are equipped to take practical, concrete actions in accordance with your decisions
- include not only caregivers but also HIV+ people who are living life to the fullest.

This means people who understand that HIV is nothing more than one of life's challenges and are prepared to support you while you are dealing with it. Despite the popular media slant on HIV infection, people are surviving and supporting survivors all around you—and you can survive, too.

ASSEMBLING YOUR MEDICAL TEAM

Who has the power to make the decisions that will determine the course of your life? If you are HIV+ and haven't become an active partner in your health-care planning but have put your fate into the hands of a doctor, your options are limited by that person's knowledge and opinions. But if you are an equal partici-pant, and if you are lucky enough to have a *team* of doctors, as opposed to a single individual, your options become more abun-dant, and so do your chances for survival.

Consider this: Over the ten years since the HIV pandemic began, predictions about its future course have been proved wrong time after time. Projected figures have had to be revised, and revised again. When the future grows this uncertain, conser-vatism sets in. Like the vast majority of human beings, many health-care providers have been unwilling to take chances in developing innovative treatment regimens or making treatment decisions on a case-by-case basis. Instead, they devise a cautious approach and stick with it. So if an HIV+ person walks in the door, doctors of this type prescribe the same treatments they prescribed for all their other HIV+ patients. Lawsuits have over-whelmed the medical industry, and doctors make their decisions largely in terms of protecting *their* futures, not just yours.

Other doctors, however, have been fired up by the pandemic to move beyond formulaic responses and learn about *all* available treatments that could potentially be life-extending and life-saving. Do you know whether your physician is one of these self-educators? Here are some questions to help you determine whether your doctor is making treatment decisions in *your* best interests, not his or hers alone:

• Would your current doctor sit down with you and inform you about not just one course of action but a range of options and possibilities?

- Would your doctor welcome information *you* might bring into the office?
- Does your doctor explain your blood results fully and clearly?
- Does your doctor explain *why* he or she is prescribing medications and tell you what effects and side effects might result?
- Does your doctor answer your questions clearly, in lay terms, and in a respectful—not a condescending—manner?
- Does your doctor lay out information and ask you to make choices, or does he or she simply lay down the law?

Although you're assuming your provider agrees with you that it's better to be alive than dead, that person might be acting on the premise that it's better to be safe than sorry. The better-safe-than-sorry approach may give the doctor a sense of security, but it limits your options, and could limit your life as well.

I ran across a prime example of the better-safe-than-sorry approach during a recent consultation with a well-known Hollywood celebrity. He had been on the drug AZT for more than two years and was obviously failing to respond (I discuss AZT resistance at length in Chapter 10, Antiviral Options). Now, here was a very famous person—I'll call him "John"—able to afford the very best medical treatment money can buy.* His doctor, aware of his accountability not only to John but to John's public, was overly cautious in his treatment decisions. Instead of taking John off the AZT and putting him on ddI (another antiviral discussed in Chapter 10), the doctor put him on both. Early on, these two extremely toxic drugs might have been beneficial, but when one drug had already proved to be of no benefit, the wisdom of prescribing it was questionable—and in this case it was devastating. I acted quickly to remove the AZT from John's regimen, and within five days he began to improve. Unfortunately, the change came too late in this case. There was already a severe loss in immune competence and John could never regain his health. He passed away about three months later.

FULL PARTICIPATION: AN EXAMPLE

Many treatment options for HIV infection have not been fully tested but have shown effectiveness and low toxicity in conclusive preliminary trials. Others have been approved by the Food and Drug Administration for prescription but not specifically for treating conditions related to HIV infection. Conservative doctors may be unwilling to prescribe any treatments not specifically endorsed for use in treating HIV infection. So finding a doctor willing to try options, as long as their toxicity is minimal, would be most beneficial.

When Don discovered that he was HIV+, he came to me for counseling. I advised him, as I do all my clients, to begin his search for treatments by first seeking a support group and counseling, which would assist him in his search for a doctor. The first order of business was to get through the initial anxiety, recover from the experience of an HIV+ bloodwork result, and get involved with people who could identify with this issue. I also urged him to explore his insurance options thoroughly so he could secure the best possible medical treatment covered by his particular plan.

Don's first T4-cell count was 685. T4 cells (also called T cells) are the backbone of the immune system and one of the cells that HIV targets, which is why immune suppression is a distinguishing feature of HIV infection. The normal T4-cell range for non-HIV+ people is 500 to 1,500 (this is a broad approximate range, which varies from lab to lab). Although Don's count was excellent for a person infected with HIV, it did reflect some immune suppression, so I gave him detailed information on a high-dose vitamin C regimen, shown by the Linus Pauling Institute to slow HIV replication in test tube research.

Don began the vitamin therapy as well as blue-green algae, a natural marine organism reported by the *Journal of the National Cancer Institute* to stimulate organs responsible for T4-cell production. Last, in response to research results demonstrating that vitamin B_{12} deficiency contributes to the cognitive impairment related to HIV infection, Don arranged to incorporate vitamin B_{12} injections into his treatment regimen.

I noticed that Don's doctor hadn't outlined a monitoring plan of any sort and suggested that Don ask for his blood to be drawn at three-month intervals to monitor his immune status. After Don had been on the customized regimen for three months, his T_4-cell count went up to 910. Six months later his T_4 reading was 1,137, and today the cell count is 1,200—there is no sign of immune suppression. The increases in T_4 cells were probably the result of this nontoxic treatment regimen, although the increases could have been due to something else, such as Don's attitude or his increased feeling of empowerment. Had Don not taken the initiative to obtain outside counseling and information, he might never have heard of any of the treatments that proved so dramatically beneficial to him.

It was clear that Don's doctor, who happened to be HIV+ himself, had gone along with the plan mostly to humor his patient. But after watching Don improve, he discounted the regimen's responsibility for Don's progress and instead began to question whether Don had been HIV+ at all! Ironically, as long as there was immune suppression, the doctor seemed content—in fact, almost pleased—with Don's condition. But after six months, when the numbers crossed a thousand, he became hostile, telling Don that he had probably never been HIV+ at all.

Many patients would have accepted the physician's assessment as accurate. But Don saw things differently: almost in spite of his doctor, he had explored the possibilities and gained precious extra time to enjoy life. He and I both felt sorry for the physician—this doctor was so close-minded that he was becoming ill from his own condition without ever once considering the possibility that some of the treatments that had helped Don might have been effective for him as well. Nevertheless, Don's own attitude remained optimistic. "Perhaps I'll even be around when they find the cure," he said to me.

TAKING CHARGE

It was relatively easy for Don to take the initiative based on outside information, because he considered his doctor and other health-care providers to be his employees. Employers explain to employees what they expect of them and set the tone and style of the relationship. Consciously taking this self-reliant attitude instead of passively accepting your doctor's advice, which is how

Americans have been conditioned to receive medical care, will help you to:

- secure for yourself the most effective medical treatment
- achieve ongoing, clear, effective, mutually respectful two-way communication with your health-care providers—meaning that they both keep you fully informed and welcome your input
- customize a treatment regimen to your specific needs (not theirs) that is flexible enough to be changed when you learn of something new and decide you want to try it

Taking charge of your medical treatment is the first step to complete self-empowerment. Once you have decided to participate fully in your treatment choices, you may find that you attract to yourself just the information you need. You might even have all the resources you need right in front of you right now without knowing it. When you are *aware* of your needs, the solutions become evident.

TAKING THE TIME YOU NEED

I've heard many HIV+ people call their diagnosis the most transforming and illuminating experience of their lives. "It's ironic," one client told me. "It took some unknown virus to put me in charge of my life and make me realize how much I love it. There's no question that I'm living more fully and enjoying my life more than I ever did before."

People have expressed many versions of this remark to me over the last ten years. Time and again, for people diagnosed with HIV infection, what is insignificant and superficial drops away and what is important in life begins to shine clearly.

And yet if you expect this sort of profound personal transformation to take place overnight, you can risk putting added and unnecessary emotional pressure on yourself. The same is true about taking charge—becoming overly concerned, overly anxious, about striking the "right" tone, doing the "right" thing, can make you crazy. So you make a mistake—you can fix it.

Yes, make it your goal to gain control of your medical treatment, but allow yourself the time and space to absorb the shift and to be human, with room for imperfection.

SOME CONCRETE SUGGESTIONS

The first step toward taking charge is working on your attitude. But there are some practical steps you can take to increase your sense of control:

• Carry a notebook with you everywhere and write down anything and everything you hear and see that might possibly apply to your medical situation now or in the future. Also, write down all your questions and take the list to your doctor's office. Record any information you hear in conversation with others, on the radio, on television, or see in newspapers, books, magazines, or other sources. Information is your greatest friend—don't trust your note-taking to memory: *write everything down.*

• If you feel anxious or uncertain about your ability to assert yourself, role-play your medical visits ahead of time. Have someone in your support group or someone who has agreed to be your sounding board take the part of your doctor, while you practice asking questions and making your wishes known.

• If you say something to your doctor that you regret, apologize and keep trying until you get it right. The medical world may be new to you; it takes practice to learn your way around it. You'll never learn how to phrase things if you don't practice, and you'll never figure anything out if you don't ask questions and keep on asking until you understand. Let your doctor know that you're not being critical when you ask questions but that you're just trying to understand so you can participate actively in your medical care. If your doctor seems impatient or annoyed by your efforts to ask questions or explain yourself, try your best to make your ideas clear. Remember, finding a new doctor is always an option. You don't have to put up with a lot of negative interactions with your health-care provider.

SELF-EMPOWERMENT SAVES LIVES

Self-empowerment contributes to your emotional well-being, but that's not why I'm spending so much space on it here. *Self-empowerment doesn't just make you feel better psychologically; it contributes to the physical healing process and saves lives.* In the book *Surviving AIDS,** author Michael Callen looks at what long-term AIDS survivors have in common and identifies seven characteristics in those people he interviewed who had survived their diagnosis, some for up to ten years. "Survivors tend to have extraordinary relationships with their health care providers," writes Callen. "Survivors spoke of a healing partnership with their health care providers, and were neither passively compliant nor defiant."

Bernie Siegel, M.D., in his best-selling book *Love, Medicine, and Miracles,* also explores the qualities shared by long-term survivors of life-threatening disease, in this case cancer. One quality that emerges above all is *fight*—the fierce determination to live. The people Siegel sees as surviving cancer are those whom health-care providers often perceive as "difficult patients" (Siegel calls them "exceptional patients"). These people:

- ask a lot of questions
- challenge their doctors' decisions
- and bring outside information to their doctors' attention.

To some health-care providers, people with these traits might indeed seem "difficult," but to me these people are self-empowered—doing all they can to take care of themselves. Self-empowered patients don't argue for the sake of argument or engage in power struggles to prove their strength. Instead, they do whatever is necessary to get the best care—researching the options, evaluating and bringing in information, and finally making informed personal decisions. And, as Bernie Siegel has shown very persuasively, these patients' full participation and stubborn determination contribute to their survival.

---

* For publisher information on most books cited in text, you can refer to the book list in Chapter 20, A Resource Guide.

GUIDELINES FOR HIRING A HEALTH-CARE PARTNER

Step 1 toward self-empowerment is to go inward and search your soul for the strength to take control through support groups, meditation, and spiritual self-awareness.

Step 2 is to turn outward and ask some specific practical questions, notebook in hand. Here are the questions you need to start with:

What options does your insurance offer you?

Here's a brief survey of the available kinds of health insurance:

• *Government insurance programs* (e.g., Medicaid, MediCal)— Your choices under these plans are more limited in some states than others. Under government insurance programs, comprehensive medical care is usually provided through hospital clinics. It makes sense to call your local community-based AIDS organization for information on the clinics in your area. With all the information in front of you, you may see that you can exercise choice in where to go for treatment.

• *Medicare*—This option is available to many on disability. Medicare is accepted by many more private doctors than are the other government-funded insurance programs.

• *HMOs* (Health Maintenance Organizations)—The options under HMOs can be more limiting than those under state and federal insurance programs. HMOs maintain networks of doctors that you must choose from, and often the best choices for HIV+s are not included on these lists. In addition, the HMO program decides what medical procedures it will pay for, whereas under other plans it is the doctor who makes the choices. Finally, HMOs don't pay for many of the "fringe" treatments for HIV (that is, experimental or alternative treatments) that the other plans regularly reimburse.

• *Private insurance* (e.g., Blue Cross, Blue Shield, 80-percent-deductible programs)—These are the best choice for HIV+s. They provide the most varied choices of qualified HIV professionals and treatment options. And if you need to go on state disability, most states allow you to keep your private insurance as long as you pay the premiums. (This plan of paying the premiums while out on disability is called COBRA in New York state; each state has a different plan, so call your local HIV organization for additional information.)

Next, track down some referrals to doctors from friends and community health resources, and prepare yourself to grill them until you're satisfied with what you hear, and feel comfortable about working with them.

What should you ask in interviewing potential doctors?

• The personal interview, either by phone or in person, is the most important part of your search for a health-care partner. When you have read the other chapters in this book, you'll have come up with your own list of questions geared to your specific needs. *Write those questions in your notebook.* You'll be amazed at what you can forget once you're face-to-face with a doctor in that examining room.

Pay careful attention to how the person responds to your questions. If the doctor decides you're a "difficult patient"—meaning a pain in the ass—you're going to treat that as a serious red flag. And if, in your initial meeting, the doctor responds with defensiveness rather than respectful answers, there's no reason to assume that things will get any better between you.

Is the doctor cold and curt? Is he or she acting superior and making you feel helpless and useless? Or do you feel the doctor is caring, attentive, and interested in you as a person? Gut instinct is all you can go on here—but it's really all you need.

• Take out your notebook and ask about specifics—for example, "I read about immune modulators. Do you prescribe them? Which ones?" Write down the answers, but pay attention, too, to the doctor's attitude toward your questions. It's a bad sign if the doctor responds with a "Now, now, why not let *us* take care of that."

• Pay particular attention to the information in this book (in Chapter 5) on interpreting your own bloodwork. Then ask the doctor you are interviewing which blood tests he or she generally relies on. If they do not compare with the tests discussed in this book, ask if the doctor is willing to order those. If the answer is no, ask why.

• Most important, ask if the doctor is open to trying new options. Does the doctor have a general approach? If you totally disagree with the regimen described or if you come up with ideas or information on your own, will the doctor prescribe other options and continue to monitor you? Some physicians refuse care if a patient tries an alternative approach. Such practitioners will insist on sticking to the regimen they know even if you fail to respond to it. If your doctor is one of those, you would be much better off with someone who knows less but is open to reading and learning.

• Does your doctor treat you with respect at all times? HIV infection is hard enough; nobody needs the added stress of a difficult and painful relationship with a physician or other caregiver. The unknowns of HIV stimulate fears and put tremendous pressures on everyone—care providers as well as patients and their loved ones. By no means are all providers defensive and disrespectful, but enough HIV+ people have had negative medical experiences to make the quality of the doctor-patient relationship an issue of concern. If a health-care provider treats you with disrespect, take comfort from the knowledge that the extra effort required to find a new person will be more than worthwhile in terms of emotional ease. And be assured that even within the most conservative medical establishment, it is possible to find caring professionals who understand the crucial importance of mutual respect.

Remember, too, that medical opinion is just that—*opinion*, often based on limited, unsubstantiated information. Despite the tone of authority your doctor might assume in prescribing treatments or discussing the course of your infection, wherever possible get a second, third, even fourth opinion, whether from another doctor or through the information resources you have come to trust (including this book; see in particular Chapter 20, A Resource Guide*).

It's a good idea to try to choose a doctor who works in an environment with others. Not only can partners monitor each other's practice, but they can potentially introduce each other to new ideas and information.

---

* Chapter 20 is a comprehensive resource guide including information on HIV- and AIDS-related organizations, treatment services, further reading, and more; it is referred to throughout this book as the Resource Guide.

Although having a care team is most beneficial, it is advisable to have one doctor you trust coordinating all decisions within the care team. In addition, a doctor who knows your medical history thoroughly can make decisions based on that history that might affect your treatment choices. For instance, a patient with allergies to certain drugs would benefit from having a physician who was well aware of this condition. Obviously, the less familiar a physician is with a patient's history, the more important it is for the patient to provide that doctor with all relevant information, such as drug allergies.

• Ask the doctor if he or she would mind asking one or two patients to call you. It's against medical ethics for the doctor to give you patients' names, but it's not a breach of confidentiality to have a patient call you on your request. Ask the doctor's patients about the services the doctor provides. Many people respond very candidly when their opinion is asked, and any patient who takes the trouble to respond to your call for information will no doubt do so in the spirit of helpfulness. The waiting room is also a good place to ask other patients for their candid opinions of the doctor.

Before hospitalization, find out about the hospital your doctor is affiliated with. Specifically, does the hospital have a good reputation for and a lot of experience in treating people with HIV infection?

Many people are surprised to learn that some hospitals have no experience at all in treating HIV-infected patients (some even have an unstated policy of refusing treatment to HIV+ patients). If you wind up in a facility like that, you may find out too late that the staff lacks insight into and an understanding of HIV infection and the latest strategies of care. Even if your doctor is aware of all current treatments, try to anticipate what would happen if a decision had to be made in the hospital when your doctor was unavailable. It's important that you be cared for by HIV-literate professionals who have had experience in dealing with HIV infection every day.

You might even want to visit the hospital and talk with an HIV+ patient. It shouldn't be that hard to find somebody who is willing or even glad to talk with you—as you've probably already noticed, a bond can form quickly between strangers who share the experience of HIV infection. Besides, HIV+ people are generally happy for visitors. But if the idea of starting a conversation cold makes you uncomfortable, try to arrange a visit through an HIV community agency (see the listings in the Resource Guide at the end of this book).

Or you might just go to the hospital and watch how the staff treats the HIV+ patients there. Usually, those patients are all together on one floor or in one wing of the hospital. Hospitals are depressing enough under the best of circumstances, so it's important to make sure HIV patients are not treated with unnecessary precautions, fear, and ignorance. Pay attention to the following—and trust your gut reactions:

• Do nurses and other workers come into the rooms? Even health-care workers can be ignorant of how the virus is transmitted, and you could find out that nurses and aides are afraid to step in the door, sometimes offering patients services from the hall.

• Do staff suit up unnecessarily with special gowns, masks, and gloves to protect against contaminants that do not exist?

• Are food trays left outside the room by the door?

• Are staff friendly and caring or distant, cold, and over-cautious?

• Is the hospital clean and inviting?

• Are there windows, television sets, and visitors' chairs in the rooms?

• Is the hospital easily accessible to the people you'll want near you? Are visiting hours long enough? Some hospitals have stingy hours; others are more relaxed. Some hospital personnel discourage visitors in underhanded ways—by expressing irritation through body language or interrupting personal conversations—even while the hospital policies are fairly liberal. Visitors are important to your emotional and physical recovery. Letting visitors in means letting *love* in—and as everyone who has ever set foot in a hospital knows, there are times when love is the strongest medicine of all. Find out whether the hospital will permit that "love medicine" to find you in the form of phone calls, visitors, and a general atmosphere of friendly concern.

• Do you sense discrimination against gays in the atmosphere?

• To the best of your ability, can you tell if the staff judges IV (intravenous) drug users harshly?

• Do you sense discrimination against HIV+ people?

You'll need to rely largely on your intuition for answers to these last questions. The bottom line is your comfort and gut-level trust in the care. If you feel unwelcome, you may need to search for another doctor whose hospital affiliations inspire more confidence and ease. Or ask your doctor if he or she has a colleague who can admit you to another hospital where you feel more comfortable.

This interview procedure might seem like a long haul, but the result will be trust and mutual understanding between your doctor and yourself. If you listen to your heart as well as your mind, you'll be opening the possibility for you and your doctor to explore all possible options in customizing treatment to your needs. And both of you will be able to proceed on the assumption that anything is possible—not only many symptom-free years, but full, complete remission or healing.

Today, many health-care professionals, including myself, consider HIV infection to be a manageable chronic illness. Treatments exist *now* for slowing the progression of HIV infection. Anyone who tells you differently is walking down the one road you don't need to travel. With an HIV+ status, you have no time to wait and everything to gain from discovering and exploring all paths that could potentially lead to what you need: your healing.

IS SPENDING TIME WITH YOUR DOCTOR GOOD MEDICINE?

How do you feel when you leave your doctor's office? Do you go home and cry after a doctor's visit? Do you go to three or four support-group meetings per week to counteract the negative messages your health-care professional hands you? And is the week before your next appointment like a chair lift to high anxiety?

The medical community acknowledges that stress has a role in activating HIV infection. Yet many health professionals do nothing to alleviate the stress associated with the condition, and many carelessly or unknowingly exacerbate that stress in a hundred different avoidable ways. Would it be so difficult to take five minutes to explain test results in clear language and a supportive, nonthreatening, nonjudgmental, and, above all, nonfatalistic tone?

Too many caregivers leave their everyday style of social interaction at home and, in their practices, limit their talk to statistics and theories. But statistics and theories do not help people—and they often elicit fear and frustration.

Most of the information ingested by the medical establishment is generated by drug companies, which have a large vested interest in promoting their products. That means that the information they disseminate in their promotional literature is often by nature slanted to favor a certain product. For example, information on superior products from other companies is never mentioned in a competitive manufacturer's advertising and promotion for obvious reasons. By believing and passing on this information, members of the medical establishment end up feeling helpless, hopeless, fearful, and defeated—and that's before you ever walk into the office.

Let me give you some examples of the effect of this negativity on doctor-patient interactions involving specific individuals (note: *individuals,* not statistics).

Case 1: Jack is HIV+ and asymptomatic. His T-cell count is 900, a good, strong number. His doctor diagnoses him with a skin condition called seborrhea and says, "Well, this is HIV-related and happens to a lot of people who are HIV positive. You're lucky it's not all over your face."

The fact is, Jack has had dry skin all his life. His seborrhea *may* be HIV-related, but with 900 T cells, there's a good chance that it is not.

And was the comment about "all over your face" absolutely necessary? That only gives Jack a detail he would never have thought of to worry about every morning when he looks in the mirror.

Case 2: Karen is HIV+. From her routine bloodwork, her doctor makes a diagnosis of a type of bone cancer. On hearing the diagnosis, Karen becomes scared, withdrawn, and depressed. Her doctor sends her to a specialist, who tells her that her practitioner failed to perform the proper tests to confirm such a diagnosis—and says that in fact he doesn't believe she has bone cancer at all. Guess how Karen feels. "Confused" is just the beginning of a description of her state of mind.

The back-and-forth shuffle between doctors can make a patient feel trapped in a nightmare, especially if those doctors have conflicting opinions. Any medical practitioner who is incapable of diagnosing or handling a situation should refer the patient to another doctor without adding his or her personal opinions to the stew. It doesn't take a lot of empathy, just a little—along with a bit of respect—to realize that casual remarks about life-threatening matters are bound to cause emotional pain.

Case 3: David has remained healthy for six years with HIV infection. His T4 cells range between 700 and 800. He runs into his primary-care physician at a dinner party. "David," says the doctor, "how are you doing? Everything all right?"

"I'm kind of upset," he tells the doctor. "My T4 cells have dropped since I saw you last."

"Well," says the doctor before turning away to another conversation, "that was bound to happen sooner or later."

At these words, David feels sick—and he wonders, is he sick with fear or is he feeling the effects of the infection? It doesn't take long for him to make his excuses and leave. The sleepless night he spends with his doctor's words echoing in his mind turns out to be the first in a long stretch of insomnia, which makes him feel worse by the day and only fuels his anxiety.

These and a thousand other examples of thoughtlessness prompt me to take this opportunity to address the medical community directly. I write from the point of view of an HIV+ person who has detected a strain of negativity running through his or her physician's communications. If you are in a situation where you feel this step is necessary, you might want to reproduce this letter and hand it (or mail it anonymously) to your own medical caregiver:

Dear Doctor,

We are people with HIV. Please talk to us with consideration for our emotions and respect for our intelligence. The patient/doctor relationship is a partnership, and our cooperation is essential for carrying out the treatments you prescribe. Why alienate us with your choice of words and tone of voice?

Many training programs for medical practitioners now exist that focus on developing the skills necessary for communicating with HIV-infected people. Perhaps, if you are unsure about the language and tone to use in conveying information to us, you might look into one of these.

In requesting empathy on your part, we are not asking to be

misled. We are asking for accurate, solution-oriented responses that explore, rather than limit, the full range of options and possibilities. Further, we are asking that you come to terms with the fact that many people are surviving with HIV and AIDS.

We know a lot of survivors. Maybe you should make an effort to meet some, too.

Sincerely,

BREAKING THE MYTHS

Myth: Most medical practitioners know about all the treatment options appropriate for HIV infection and are willing to prescribe them.
Truth: If you follow the interview process recommended in this chapter, you'll find out that medical professionals' knowledge and experience range from next to none to a great deal. Those who went to school before the pandemic may know very little about HIV infection.

Myth: Because of their training, doctors see medical situations more clearly than other people do.
Truth: Doctors are human beings with the same foibles as the rest of us.

Myth: Because of their training, doctors are more compassionate and empathetic than other people.
Truth: Medical schools rarely look at and seldom teach their students to pay attention to the emotional experiences of patients.

Myth: Older doctors are wiser than younger ones, since they have more experience.
Truth: Younger doctors have done their residencies in the age of HIV infection and often have a lot of practical experience with HIV.

Questions You Need Answered

- What kind of insurance coverage do you have?
- What medical and support services are available to you under that coverage?
- What kinds of services are available in your community—for example, community-based AIDS organizations?
- How can you use those community services to help you choose your medical team?
- How comfortable do you feel with the doctor or doctors you are considering?
- How comfortable do they seem to feel with you—and with your full participation in your own treatment?
- What hospital is your doctor or doctors associated with?
- What are your options if you don't feel comfortable there?
- What are your alternatives if things don't work out with the medical team you settle on?
- Can you change insurance carriers if you feel other coverage would offer more options? (Some jobs offer a choice of HMOs and private insurance)
- How do you get a listing of support services and groups in your area?

CHAPTER 2

HIV: An Overview

To design and manage a treatment regimen effectively, and to modify that treatment down the line if necessary, it's important that you understand how the HIV virus functions.

Still, I have mixed feelings about sharing this information.

The emotional environment of your body can severely affect your healing, and all of us have taken in enough negative information about HIV infection to last three lifetimes—we don't need to ingest more. But if you change the way you perceive and process the information that comes your way, your feelings about the data itself could change and its impact on your emotional state would therefore be minimized. Here's what I mean:

• Whenever you hear a negative statement about HIV, remind yourself that it is not necessarily true for *you*. Each person is different, and HIV manifests itself differently in every infected person.

• Every time you hear a statistic, remind yourself that you are not a number on a chart and that statistics do not apply to everyone. For every statistic that exists about HIV infection, there is someone who has defied that number.

• Don't be snowed by credentials. Despite the fact that there are many scientists and medical professionals going around making pronouncements and predictions about the future, remind yourself that such statements are empty words, not facts. A statement such as "everyone with HIV will get sick" is a theoretical opinion, *not a proven fact.*

• HIV is one of the most unpredictable, inconsistent conditions we have worked with. Remember, people are living with an AIDS diagnosis they received ten years ago and more. Michael Callen, who wrote about his personal experience in *Surviving AIDS,* is just one of the many who have defied the statistics. Remind yourself that you are not a statistic; you are an individual who can break any mold.

• Remain focused on the fact that there are many treatment options available to help stop the progression of HIV. You might feel that you already know more about HIV than you ever wanted to know; but the more information you gather, the more ammunition you will have for conquering this virus.

That said, I can begin to help you arm yourself by discussing how HIV functions.

WORD ONE: CONTROVERSY

HIV, human immunodeficiency virus, is the virus most scientists believe causes the disease called AIDS, or acquired immunodeficiency syndrome. There is some controversy over whether this virus alone can cause AIDS, or even whether the virus is the cause of AIDS at all. In studying the way HIV works in the body, both in my practice and in the scientific literature, I have concluded that HIV is a major contributing factor in the development of the disease AIDS. Although there are still only theories on the action of HIV, two of these theories seem supported by most of the evidence. What follows is an exploration of these theories.

It is believed that the HIV virus causes two kinds of damage at the cellular level:

• It interferes with normal cell function and sparks an autoimmune dysfunction in a bodily function called *apoptosis,* in which the cells destroy themselves.
• It destroys cells by infecting them directly.

Important Characteristics of HIV

- HIV is a small, simple virus.
- It's a relatively weak virus.
- Two things make HIV difficult to control:
    1) the "docking arms" (see diagram, page 29) on the virus that allow it access to cells and permit it to undermine the very system designed to control it;
    2) some viruses change appearance, preventing the immune system from identifying them.

Many of the cells affected by the virus are important to the proper functioning of the immune system. In the past, when a significant number of cells in the body have been damaged or destroyed by HIV, the resulting conditions have been collectively referred to as:

- AIDS, or acquired immunodeficiency syndrome,
- or ARC (AIDS-related complex).

But distinguishing between these two terms has become problematic. Increasingly, all the conditions resulting from the presence of the virus within the body are denoted by the single term

- *HIV disease or infection.*

COFACTORS

Certain conditions, called cofactors, may exacerbate the action of HIV within the human body. However, our information about these cofactors and their impact on the progression of HIV infection is new and sketchy, and research to date has been minimal. Because of the danger of mistaking speculation and hypothesis for scientific fact, I feel it's important for us to concentrate our efforts on the processes for which we have the most evidence and to deal with cofactors that substantial research findings have revealed.

This decision reflects my attitude in general. In this book, as in my work in counseling HIV+ people and designing their treatment regimens, I am concerned with the interventions supported by the greatest amount of research. Speculations, possibilities, rumors, and fantasies are fine if you are healthy and able to monitor their efficacy. But we already have a great deal of information about HIV, so let's get started.

THE STRUCTURE OF HIV

The human immunodeficiency virus, like all viruses, is composed mostly of protein. Each virus is a round ball of protein studded with protuberances commonly referred to as *docking arms.* These "arms" are actually molecules of a protein called gp-120, and they greatly determine how the virus infects, damages, and destroys healthy cells in the body (see Figure 2-1).

Other proteins, as well as a layer of lipid (fat) molecules, are also found on the virus's outer surface, but understanding the significance and function of gp-120, the docking arm, in particular will help you understand how certain treatments work.

Located inside the viral sphere is the *viral core.* Its contents are essential to the replication of the virus and become active only once HIV has infected a human cell.

As you read about the way HIV infects a cell, refer to Figure 2-2.

INFECTION: WHAT IT IS

One of the best-supported theories as to the way HIV infects a cell is the viral infection theory. The process of infection begins when HIV attaches to a cell—called a *host cell*—in the body. This attachment process takes place by means of the virus's docking arms, composed of gp-120. These "arms" fit the "sleeves" of another protein, CD4, which is found on the surface of some cells. When the viral arm slips into the CD4 sleeve, virus and cell are bonded together.

HIV cannot bond with cells that lack CD4 on their surface. Many cells in the immune system *do* have the crucial surface component—T-helper or T4 cells, for example. Also, some cells in the brain, lungs, lower intestinal tract, and bone marrow have surface CD4.

Once bonded to a cell, the HIV penetrates the cell's membrane,

FIGURE 2-1   The HIV Virus

The viral core, made mostly of RNA, is protein 24 (P24). The protein gp-120 makes up the "docking arms" that the HIV virus uses to infect cells.

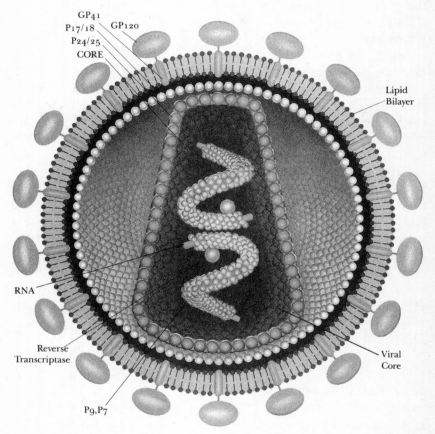

GP41
P17/18   GP120
P24/25
CORE

Lipid Bilayer

RNA

Reverse Transcriptase

Viral Core

P9,P7

or surface. At this point, the virus's own shell dissolves and its contents, the viral core, is left inside the cell.

Although HIV infects many kinds of cells in the body—and in that way causes dysfunction—its action in T4 cells is most heavily documented and has the most far-reaching effects on bodily function.

RNA is the main constituent of the viral core. It contains the virus's *genetic code*, which enables HIV to make copies of itself. Also contained in the viral core are three enzymes, substances that trigger biochemical processes:

- reverse transcriptase
- integrase
- protease

Once inside the T4 cell, these three enzymes, along with the viral RNA, enter the host cell's *nucleus,* which houses the cell's *DNA*—genetically coded instructions that control the cell's functions.

Inside the host cell's nucleus, the invading reverse transcriptase begins to convert HIV's RNA into DNA.

Integrase, another of the enzymes, causes the virus's newly converted DNA to attach to the host cell's DNA—which changes the genetic instructions governing the cell's activities. This completes the infection of the host cell.

Many promising treatments work to interrupt infection on a cellular level. For example, dextran sulfate* theoretically interferes with the ability of the gp-120 and CD4 proteins to bond together. Another treatment floods the body with free-floating CD4 to bond with all the viral docking arms before they connect with cellular CD4. (Like other drugs, the one used in this treatment is named for the cell material it mimics—in this case, CD4.) AZT, on the other hand, interrupts the function of reverse transcriptase, thus interfering with the reproductive ability of HIV. Keeping the principles of HIV cell infection clearly in your mind will help you understand the function of other treatment options described in this book.

THE RETROVIRUS

HIV is smaller and weaker than other viruses, but its most distinctive feature is that it is a *retrovirus.* Most viruses known to infect humans already contain DNA when they invade a cell and do not need reverse transcriptase to reproduce their genetic code. The fact that HIV's core of RNA, rather than the "normal" DNA, uses reverse transcriptase to reproduce marks it as a retrovirus. Scientists have known of retroviruses infecting animals since the beginning of the century, but not until 1980 was a

---

* Drugs have scientific, generic names as well as the brand names given to them by their manufacturers. In Part II of this book, when I discuss treatment options, I list the brand name first and then the generic name.

retrovirus discovered that infected human beings. This retrovirus was HIV.

DORMANCY AND THE INFECTION TIME LINE

In most cases, cells infected with HIV continue their normal
activities, even reproducing as before. Some researchers believe
that in some cases, infection will not advance beyond this point.
This state is called dormancy. At worst, such people's cell function
could be slightly impaired, but for the most part cells function
normally.

Other researchers believe that everyone infected with HIV will
eventually get sick. This is not a fact but a theoretical projection—
one of those dangerously abstract intellectual constructions I
warned against earlier—based on incomplete statistics. Also,
these statistics represent untreated cases—people in whom no
medical or alternative treatments were used. Instead of project-
ing, I prefer the truth:

- We still don't know the way HIV infection runs its course.
- A recent study shows that 11 percent of the people infected
  with HIV for ten years or more, and some without the benefit
  of treatment interventions, show no sign of HIV progression
  or symptoms (no abnormal bloodwork or HIV-related infections).
- Research on HIV infection is new and inconclusive, and statistics differ tremendously from source to source.

Don't allow yourself to get hung up on numbers. Remember, we
are all individuals, and one of the characteristics of HIV is that it
reacts differently in each person it infects. The course of events
following infection can be serious—there is no disputing that. But
I firmly believe that with a thorough knowledge of interventions it
is possible to interrupt, contain, and control the virus.

If your health-care provider makes predictions about time periods and "factual" statements regarding HIV progression, be-
ware! Cut-and-dried, "definitive" statements made without a
"maybe" or a "possibly" can be extremely damaging to your
emotional state—and keeping your psyche as well as your body
strong and healthy is fundamental to the management of this

infection. It's common sense to keep your spirit and body strong in the face of a challenge to your health. Anyone who undermines your emotional strength, thoughtlessly or otherwise, by insisting on unproven "facts" needs to be counted out.

The only accurate facts are these:

- We don't know how long progression will take.
- We don't know if or when infected people will get sick.
- We don't know who will get sick.
- We have some indicators that can help us make predictions, but these indicators are not foolproof.

As a matter of fact, the only virus known to cause symptoms in every person it infects is rabies. Some of us believe that there are HIV-infected people who will never develop symptoms—and this belief is completely justifiable, given the existing facts.

As I write this, many, many HIV+ people with supposedly poor bloodwork results are symptom-free and feeling well. It's been a habit of the medical establishment and the mainstream press to ignore these individuals or to treat them as very rare exceptions. My goal is to bring those people to your attention as often as I can, answering negativity with the facts.

HOW THE VIRUS REPRODUCES

Once infection is no longer dormant, new particles of HIV begin to assemble within the host cell. How precisely this happens is not yet clear, though scientists do know that the third enzyme contained in the viral core, protease, is necessary to the process. Researchers are currently seeking ways of interrupting the function of protease in the same way that AZT interrupts the function of reverse transcriptase.

Once assembled within the cell, the new pieces of HIV push out the membrane of the infected cell, forming buds. Eventually these buds break off. These new cells of HIV destroy the host cell and migrate through the body to infect other cells (see Figure 2-2).

This series of steps is known as viral progression. As with other viruses, HIV can reproduce in this way and possibly lead to illness. But HIV might also spark a process known as apoptosis, a more recent discovery. Apoptosis is a function of the body in

FIGURE 2-2   **Viral Reproduction**

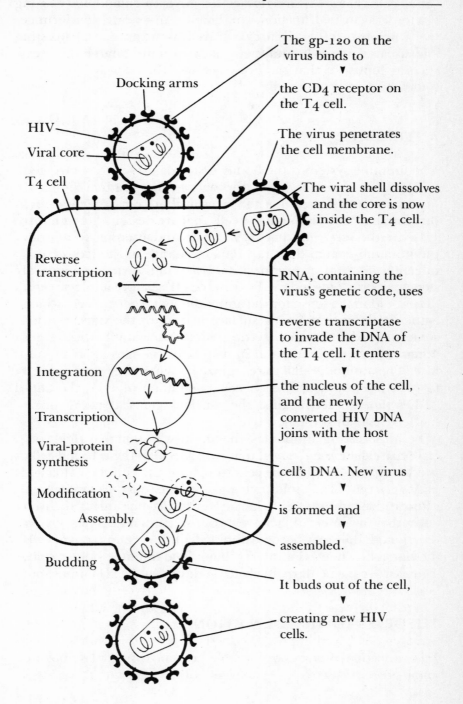

The gp-120 on the virus binds to ▾

the CD4 receptor on the T4 cell.

Docking arms

The virus penetrates the cell membrane.

HIV

Viral core

The viral shell dissolves and the core is now inside the T4 cell.

T4 cell

Reverse transcription

RNA, containing the virus's genetic code, uses ▾

reverse transcriptase to invade the DNA of the T4 cell. It enters ▾

Integration

the nucleus of the cell, and the newly converted HIV DNA joins with the host ▾

Transcription

Viral-protein synthesis

cell's DNA. New virus ▾

Modification

Assembly

is formed and ▾

assembled.

Budding

It buds out of the cell, ▾

creating new HIV cells.

which cells that are no longer needed are eliminated. HIV causes this process to malfunction, sparking an autoimmune dysfunction whereby useful cells are destroyed in the apoptosis process. This is similar to what happens in other autoimmune diseases, such as lupus, in that the body actually turns on its own cells somehow destroying them.

ANTIBODIES

The immune system is the bodily system most severely targeted by HIV, and in people with symptoms it is the gradual disabling of the immune system, not the virus itself, that can become life-threatening. Still, although the cells that are designed to fight off HIV are the very cells that HIV attacks and attempts to destroy, the immune system does not remain passive in the face of this infection. Instead, it produces *antibodies* to the virus—chemical substances custom-designed to disable HIV before it infects cells.

It would make sense for the antibodies to target gp-120, which is the single distinguishing surface feature of the virus, but for some unknown reason they do not. Instead, antibodies target other surface materials, and in response the virus alters its surface. The antibodies fail to recognize the virus they were created to neutralize, and with each new generation of HIV, the antibodies that worked against the previous generation can prove ineffective against the new one.

Besides making antibodies, the immune system may send special cells, called *macrophages,* to isolate and kill HIV-infected cells. But because these immune cells, too, have CD4 on their surface, HIV's gp-120 "arms" find their way into the cells' protein sleeves, causing the immune cells themselves to become infected. Even when they are infected, however, macrophages do not necessarily die, though they may become disabled. Only certain types of cells die outright when HIV infects them. The immune helper cells, T4 cells, are particularly likely to be destroyed by HIV infection.

THEORIES OF HIV DEPLETION

HIV infection destroys vulnerable cells in three ways that we know of:

• A large number of buds pushing out the membrane of the infected cell can cause the cell to rupture, which allows the new viral particles to enter the bloodstream and the host cell, in this case the T4 cell, to die.

• The virus's arms can damage cells by bumping into them. The body eliminates these damaged cells.

• The virus can secure itself onto several cells at once, making a cluster. Whenever the gp-120 docking arms on the HIV cell come into contact with the CD4 on another cell, bonding takes place. Together, the merged cells are called a *syncytium*; their original functions end and eventually these clusters are eliminated, as are all dysfunctional cells.

APOPTOSIS

The theories of HIV depletion described above have been extensively researched. However, although HIV infects T4 cells, the number of those cells infected by the virus has not seemed high enough to cause the T4-cell depletion seen in AIDS. It is true that the rising virus levels seen in HIV progression have suggested

---

How HIV Infects a Cell

• The protein gp-120 on the virus's surface bonds with CD4, another protein on the surface of some cells in the body.

• The virus penetrates the cell membrane.

• The outer part of the virus, called the viral shell, dissolves, leaving the viral core within the cell.

• The virus's RNA enters the cell's nucleus along with the enzymes reverse transcriptase, integrase, and protease.

• Reverse transcriptase converts the virus's RNA into DNA.

• Integrase bonds the viral DNA to the cell's DNA, changing the genetic code that governs the activities of the cell.

• Normal or slightly impaired cell function continues for years, and perhaps throughout the person's normal life span. This period is called dormancy.

• Following dormancy, the infected cell ruptures, releasing new viruses into the bloodstream.

viral infection, but recently cell depletion due to a process known as apoptosis has been observed.

During apoptosis, a cell produces an enzyme that destroys that cell's own nucleus. This process is the body's own "house cleaning," in which cells no longer useful are eliminated. The theory that apoptosis goes awry when HIV is present would suggest an auto-immune phenomenon, in which healthy T4 cells attack themselves, rather than a viral infection. The theory that apoptosis is responsible for T4-cell depletion is currently being verified by other scientific observations. In addition, new documentation suggests that nutrient and enzyme levels play a role in HIV progression. It is known that a low level of one enzyme, glutathione, makes cells vulnerable to apoptosis.

It is becoming increasingly common to gear treatment to cover both possible modes of T4-cell depletion. Anyone using natural interventions as well as many MDs suggest the use of NAC, a derivative of the amino acid cysteine, to raise glutathione levels in order to prevent apoptosis. (For more on NAC and other natural interventions, see Chapter 8.)

THE LIFE SPAN OF THE VIRUS

Inside the body the HIV virus is difficult to control, but outside the body it's easily eliminated by hot, soapy water or bleach. The virus will die quickly when exposed to air, but viruses in a droplet or pool of blood or in a syringe will live longer.

There are no studies telling us how long the virus might live in an environment unexposed to air, so it's important not to take any chances. I had a client, an IV needle user, who injected heroin and left the used needle in his parents' bathroom. About twelve hours later, his father stuck himself with the needle and became infected with HIV. This sad story isn't detailed enough to tell us much about HIV, but it does serve as a warning. Approach with caution all situations that could involve transmission of the virus. Especially if you are HIV+, be careful. As I'll explain shortly, there are good reasons why you don't want to reinfect yourself.

HOW THE VIRUS IS TRANSMITTED

In general, it's difficult to transmit the virus from one person to another. You need one of four bodily fluids to do it:

- blood
- semen (including preejaculatory fluid)
- vaginal secretions
- breast milk

Certain other bodily fluids, such as cerebral fluid, can transmit the virus as well, but they are usually omitted in lists of agents of transmission, since contact with them is rare.

In 1991, newspaper reports from the Seventh International AIDS Conference in Florence implied that saliva could transmit the virus, but this is probably untrue. Saliva can contain *particles* of HIV, but probably not enough to cause infection—clearly, if it did, the incidence of infection would be much greater. Also, the virus cannot be readily transmitted via feces, urine, or sweat; however, urine, feces, and saliva can contain blood that could transmit HIV.

The Four Bodily Fluids That Can Readily Transmit HIV

- Blood
- Semen (including preejaculatory fluid)
- Vaginal secretions
- Breast milk

- Infection can occur if one of these fluids containing the virus *enters the bloodstream.*
- The possibility of infection occurring through contact with the mucosal tissue lining of the anus/rectum, vagina, or penis is being studied.
- It is highly unlikely (and no cases have been reported) that HIV infection can be transmitted through kissing.
- Consistently practicing safer sex is most important, since one exposure can put you at risk of becoming HIV+ or reinfecting yourself with additional virus.

Infection occurs when bodily fluids containing the virus enter the bloodstream. The virus usually requires an entry point into the bloodstream for infection to occur. Definitive information on sexual transmission does not exist, and some doctors believe infection may occur by the HIV-infected bodily fluids' contact with the mucosal tissue lining of the anus/rectum, vagina, or penis. Infection can occur from a single exposure to an infected fluid, but many times an exposure does not take and infection does not occur. Since it only takes one exposure, condom use is a necessity at all times.

HIGH-RISK BEHAVIORS

Two behaviors have been identified as high-risk:

• sharing uncleaned syringes and needles
• unprotected sex

While these two are the most common transmission modes, it is possible for HIV+ mothers to transmit the virus to infants via breast milk.

First, drugs: Doing drugs isn't a great idea under any circumstances, but if you are doing injectable drugs, get a new needle and don't share it with *anyone*! Or clean your needles with straight bleach three times, then rinse with water five times.

In sexual transmission, unprotected anal intercourse holds the highest risk; unprotected vaginal intercourse comes next. Both the vagina and anal canal are lined with capillaries, and when these small blood vessels close to the surface are broken, they can serve as entry points for the virus into the bloodstream.

There are few verifiable reported cases of HIV transmission through unprotected oral sex. Unless there are open sores or cuts in the mouth, the virus is unlikely to find an entry point in the mouth—many more entry points present themselves in the vagina and anal canal via the capillaries that line both these channels. Besides, saliva seems to have a neutralizing effect on HIV (a phenomenon that we do not yet understand and that is currently under study). And if one were to swallow the virus, the acids in the stomach would in all likelihood kill it. I'm not endorsing unprotected oral sex, but facts are facts. The possibility of oral transmission exists, but the probability is much lower than with unprotected anal and vaginal intercourse.

SAFER SEX

During unprotected anal or vaginal intercourse, the inserter and recipient are at approximately equal risk of exposure to HIV, though there are reports that claim that the recipient is at higher risk. During intercourse, microscopic cuts on the penis or the vagina allow the virus access into the body. In addition, certain cells in the penis associated with the urinary tract bond with the virus and bring it into the bloodstream.

HIV infection is behavior-bound, and transmission is easy to avoid:

Use a latex barrier—a latex condom or a dental dam—during intercourse or oral sex.

That's it: that's the single principle governing safer sex.

Knowing your partner's history is not important or dependable. You can have a complete list of a person's sex partners without being sure whether they are HIV+ or not. Don't fall into the trap of "Well, this person only had one sex partner ever, so it's okay." Using a condom should be the norm. This is a behavior-bound disease, which means it doesn't matter *who* you do, it matters *what* you do. Wear a latex condom.

Using nonlatex barriers—for example, condoms made of lambskin—is not dependable. Skin condoms are porous and can allow the virus to pass through. Read the label and use *only* latex condoms, the most common type. Even protected sex with a condom has a risk because condoms can break. To add a level of protection, it is probably advisable to withdraw prior to ejaculation. (See Figure 2-3 on page 39.)

It is important to use a condom *prior* to actual genital contact, as preejaculatory fluid can contain the virus as well.

THE QUESTION OF NONOXYNOL 9

Many HIV organizations also recommend using a spermicidal lubricant containing the spermicide nonoxynol 9. It is true that nonoxynol 9 kills the virus on contact, but a Canadian study has shown that nonoxynol 9 irritates the anal and vaginal canals, causing the body to respond by rushing blood to the surface capillaries. Although not proven, the resulting theory holds that nonoxynol 9 could *increase* the likelihood of direct blood contact and therefore of HIV transmission.

Nevertheless, many people are still recommending nonoxynol 9. My recommendation is to avoid anything that might increase the likelihood of exposure. That would include nonoxynol 9.

However, do use a water-based lubricant, such as KY Jelly, to reduce friction, since friction can cause a condom to break. Never use an oil-based lubricant, such as Vaseline or other petroleum jellies—it will chemically weaken the latex.

PROTECTED SEX FOR HIV+ PEOPLE

If you are HIV+, you need to use protection—not only for the sake of your partner but for *your* sake as well. One reason is that different types of the HIV virus exist. About 90 percent of the infected people in the United States have HIV-1. In Africa, the most prevalent strain is known as HIV-2. In addition, viruses isolated from different individuals differ—scientists have identified aggressive and passive forms. HIV isolated from infected people without symptoms seems to be less aggressive than that isolated from people with HIV symptoms or AIDS. You do not want to risk adding another type or strain of virus into your body. These strains have the potential to activate other strains and types.

In addition, you do not want to increase your viral load—that is, the number of viruses in your body. Your objective is to *lower* your viral load and eliminate it. Reexposure would add to it.

For all these reasons, protect yourself from high-risk behavior. Don't exempt yourself from safer sex. Practice the safer-sex guidelines described in the box on p. 37.

A PERSONAL NOTE

I'd like to depart from the facts for a moment to inject a few personal comments on sex in the age of HIV infection. The word *abstinence* inevitably comes up in discussions of safer sex, but I do not believe anyone should consider giving up sex to avoid infection. Sex is a life-affirming process, a source of pleasure, comfort, and satisfaction that can build self-esteem and a sense of security. Safer sex alone—if it is always carefully practiced—works to prevent infection. Why sacrifice so fulfilling a source of enrichment and connection when doing so is scientifically unnecessary?

Safer-Sex Guidelines

• For intercourse and oral sex, use latex condoms, *never* ones made from animal skin. The latter are too porous and could let the virus through. Lubricated condoms are available, but for oral sex they only add a bad taste to the experience. Use nonlubricated condoms for oral sex.

• For oral vaginal sex, use latex dental dams.

• For intercourse, always use a water-based lubricant, such as KY Jelly, to prevent friction. *Never* use an oil-based lubricant (e.g., Vaseline), which could weaken condoms.

• Avoid nonoxynol 9 (see page 36).

• When using condoms (see page 39), to prevent them from breaking, make sure you
  1) leave a "reservoir tip" at the tip of the penis before you unroll the condom down the shaft so there will be room to catch the semen;
  2) release any air in the tip before rolling the condom down the shaft by lifting the base slightly and squeezing the tip.

• If you can, check the condom before ejaculating to make sure it is still intact.

• After ejaculating, men should withdraw the penis while still hard, holding the base of the condom during withdrawal to keep the semen from spilling out.

• If the condom breaks during intercourse, the man should withdraw *before* ejaculating. To add a level of protection, it is probably advisable to withdraw prior to ejaculation.

I have an HIV+ client who is a husband and father. Six years ago, around the time his child was born, he learned that he was infected with the virus. He had probably been infected several years before, when he was using intravenous drugs. Even though he and his wife had had unprotected sex for several years after his presumed infection, his wife tested HIV negative, and continues to be tested regularly. They have been practicing safer sex for six years, continuing to test HIV—every six months.

Although at one time gay men were at greatest risk for HIV infection, their adoption of safer-sex practices has slowed infection rates in this group dramatically. Today adolescents, regardless of sexual orientation, are at greatest risk of infection. We can only keep telling them, teaching them, bringing home the simple message: *safer sex prevents infection, and safer sex is protected sex, period.*

One final comment has to do with openly discussing your HIV status, especially with a lover. Most people believe that telling your lover of your status puts the relationship at risk. In my experience, when the lover is told before the first sexual encounter, this is not so. Get to know someone first, create a bond, so that when you reveal your status the other person knows and likes you for *yourself*.

People who get to know their partners before having sexual relationships find that their relationships are deeper and more meaningful, and learning that a partner is HIV+ can actually have a positive effect on an evolving relationship. It may seem strange to say it, but one thing HIV has done for us is to give our relationships new and deeper meaning. People are communicating more freely, talking out disagreements, working through problems, and making long-term commitments. If you are HIV+, I urge you to talk out your fears with your partner and encourage your partner to do the same with you.

Telling someone your fears is a very intimate act. This depth of sharing is new to many of us, but we have the chance now to relate on a level that we have all yearned to experience. If you are dating and discover that your partner is HIV+, will you run in fear or will you make a decision based on love? I'm right there with you—in my own love relationship, one of us is HIV+, one of us is not. I wouldn't trade this deeply fulfilling partnership for anything else. I have let go of fear to rely on love.

FIGURE 2-3   How to use a condom

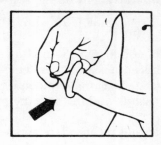

Make sure to leave a reservoir at the tip; release any air out of the tip before proceeding by lifting the rolled base slightly (see arrow) and squeezing the tip.

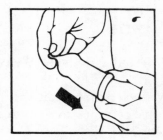

Before you roll the condom down, squeeze the tip to remove air.

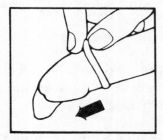

After ejaculating, withdraw the penis while still hard. Hold the rim of the condom so nothing spills while you withdraw.

Thinking about Being Tested?

• Most local departments of health provide free, anonymous HIV-antibody testing.

• Before the actual test, in a precounseling session, a counselor should explain all procedures and offer some emotional support.

• Bring a close friend to all appointments (there are usually two: the first for precounseling and the test; the second for receiving results).

• "Confidential" testing means your name is on record somewhere. I prefer anonymous testing, where only a number is used.

BREAKING THE MYTHS

Myth: Everyone infected with the HIV virus will develop HIV-related symptoms or AIDS.
Truth: We simply don't know what will happen in the long run, but many people continue to remain symptom-free while the "deadlines" come and go.

Myth: Knowing your partner's sex history is essential for safer sex.
Truth: Safer sex consists of only one principle: *use latex.*

Myth: Once you're infected, there's no reason to practice safer sex.
Truth: HIV+ people need to protect themselves against reinfection with different types and strains of the virus and to reduce, not risk increasing, the amount of virus in their bodies.

Myth: HIV can be transmitted through kissing.
Truth: Only four bodily fluids have been proven to transmit HIV—blood, semen, vaginal secretions, and breast milk. There are no reported cases of transmission through saliva.

Myth: Using nonoxynol 9 is a safer-sex practice.
Truth: Though nonoxynol 9 kills HIV on contact, there is

some evidence to suggest it can increase the risk of infection. *Avoid the risk—don't use it.*

Myth: Gay men form the largest risk group for HIV infection. **Truth:** Infection among gay men has slowed dramatically as a result of safer sex practices. The group with the highest risk now is adolescents.

CHAPTER 3

The Immune System

In the preceding chapter, I explained how the HIV virus infects immune cells, potentially weakening the body's immune response.

Can people survive with a suppressed immune system?

Maybe you'd like an emphatic yes or no to this question, but you won't get one from me—especially after the phone call I just had from an old friend in California who is dealing with AIDS as best he can.

People all over the country, people around the globe, are *doing just fine* with severely compromised immune systems. I witness this fact daily in my practice, and my friend just reinforced the point for me over the phone. He told me he felt his best when his T4-cell level was 65. Now that his T4-cell count is 250 he's grateful, but he doesn't really feel any better physically.

The body is a miraculous machine. It is designed to adapt in order to survive—and it does so sometimes in unpredictable ways. One of the best ways to become acquainted with your body as an incredible healing machine is to take a few moments to understand your immune system. If you don't know the workings of this amazing set of responses, prepare to be dazzled.

COMPONENTS OF THE IMMUNE SYSTEM

The things we call germs—microorganisms and viruses that infect our bodies and cause symptoms—are around us all the time. We drink germs, we eat them, we breathe them—we are all taking them into our bodies at what might seem an alarming rate. But once inside they are met by a formidable opponent, the immune system, and most are killed and disposed of before they ever have a chance to infect our tissues.

The immune system is made up of white blood cells, of which there are a number of distinct types, each with its own function:

• *macrophages*—cells that alert the immune system into action against an invading virus, bacteria, or toxin.

• *antibodies*—cells designed to neutralize invading viruses or the many other foreign biological substances that enter the system. Antibodies are custom-designed to match the invader's structure.

• *T4 cells (or CD4 cells, or helper cells—the terms are interchangeable; often referred to simply as T cells)*—cells that moderate the body's response to infection. Macrophages convey a chemical message to the T4 cell that an invader is present. The T4 cells determine, on the basis of the invader's structure, what an antibody to it should look like. Also, T4 cells "remember" every biological invader that ever entered the system and can respond immediately if the body has combated this particular invader before. So, if you had measles as a child, your T4 cells will respond to an invading measles virus by "recalling" the antibodies the body made for measles and producing new ones within hours. You never get measles symptoms after your initial exposure to the disease, because your immune system responds so quickly. But the first time you had measles, you developed symptoms because your body took days to create antibodies to the unfamiliar virus and bring it under control.

• *B cells*—cells that actually make the antibodies at the direction of the T4 cell.

As you can see in the accompanying diagram, this is how the cycle works:

FIGURE 3-1   The immune system

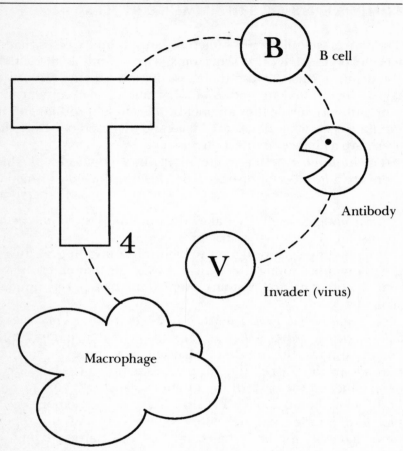

- An invader enters the body.
- The macrophage triggers the immune system into action.
- The T4 cell determines whether the invader is "familiar" and chemically signals the creation of antibodies customized to repel the invader.
- The B cells actually make the antibodies.
- The antibodies surround and neutralize the invader.
- The macrophage moves back into action to eliminate the neutralized cell from the body.
- Once the invasion is over, the T8 suppressor cells perform their function of giving a chemical signal to end the immune system's response: "All clear! Mission accomplished. Go home!"

Fantastic, no?

TESTING FOR HIV

When you get a blood test for HIV, the laboratory technicians are searching *not* for the HIV virus, but for *antibodies* to the virus. That is why a doctor might tell patients who think they have been exposed to wait for a time before being tested. It usually takes less than six months, in some cases a year, but in a small number of cases it can take more than a year for the immune system to create antibodies to HIV.

A number of factors probably account for the delay. If a person is infected through sexual contact, usually only a small amount of HIV gets into the bloodstream and causes infection. The virus may have to replicate before concentrations are high enough to alarm the body into responding to its presence. One San Francisco–based study showed that in 23 percent of the cases, HIV that was sexually transmitted took three years to show up on the regular antibody blood test. Although the data from this study has been questioned, many scientists still believe there might be a "window period" after exposure and before the body has produced antibodies.

This "window" period has a special significance when it comes to the safety of the nation's blood supply. The blood in blood banks is tested for the presence of antibodies in exactly the same way that your own blood is tested. Blood that shows no antibodies is made available to those who need transfusions for medical reasons. But the blood tested in this way may have been donated *after* exposure but *before* the production of antibodies—that is, during the "window period." So it's possible to get infected with HIV from blood that has tested negative for HIV antibodies. I encourage *all* people, whether HIV+ or not, to give blood in advance of surgery, if possible, so that it can be stored for their own use if they need it.

I am not making this recommendation to cause fear and delirium but to encourage action. The chances of dying in your car are still millions of times greater than those of getting HIV from the blood supply. But we do need to use better testing methods—already available for research—on the blood supply.

RESPONDING TO THE VIRAL LOAD

Studies tell us that when the body initially starts to make anti-bodies, the "viral load"—the number of individual viruses in the body—is high. The immune system doesn't seem to mount a response until the viral load is quite significant. But when the system *does* respond, it does so very effectively, eliminating nearly all HIV from the system.

How does the HIV virus go on to cause the symptoms? As I described earlier, one of the distinguishing characteristics of HIV is its ability to change its genetic code: the components of the virus don't change, but their structures do. Since the anti-bodies made by the immune system are specifically designed to match the genetic structure of the invading virus, when that structure changes the antibodies are unable to find their mark. So, although the immune system eliminates most of the viruses in the system, those viruses that have changed their structure escape the system's detection and go on to infect the T_4 cells—the very cells that would control them.

Now, that sounds very dramatic, very dire. So before going on I want to take a "reality break." Remember, this book is about dealing with and living with HIV infection, so let me pass on another phone story. While writing this chapter, I received a call from a client of mine who has turned his HIV progression around totally by means of an antiviral treatment described in these pages. He was having severe headaches (gone), weight and appetite loss (he can't stop eating), fatigue (he goes dancing every night), and a consistent decrease of his T_4-cell count (it has gone up by 100).

Remember:

- In many cases, HIV progression in the immune system can be reversed.
- In many cases, HIV progression can be stopped from future progression.

I would be lying if I said this was possible in every case, but in people who are not severely debilitated, successes are extremely common.

REVIEW: HOW INFECTION TAKES PLACE

Many cells in the immune system have a coat that contains receptor sites, places where other cells dock in order to communicate with the cell. Some of these receptor sites are known as CD4, a cellular protein. As I explained in Chapter 2, the virus has docking arms called gp-120 (another protein). Wherever there is CD4 in the body, gp-120 is attracted to it and fits into it like a key into a lock. According to current research, it seems that only cells with CD4 proteins on their surface can be infected by HIV.

Remember: HIV docks onto the CD4 receptor site of the T4 cell, infects the cell, and uses it as a host to produce more HIV. There are many ways to interfere with this process. By the time you finish reading this book, you will be familiar with drug treatments that do just that.

Remember, too, that once infection occurs, the virus

- may lie dormant in the cells—perhaps forever, but no one knows how long;
- may cause dysfunction;
- may destroy the cells completely.

With intervention the scenario can change completely.

LIVING WELL WITH IMMUNE SUPPRESSION

When HIV infects a T4 cell, it lives within it—sometimes for long periods, and quite possibly indefinitely. The virus merges with the cell and becomes part of it, so now you have an immune cell with a human immunodeficiency virus living inside and off of it, as a parasite does. Aside from the medical interventions discussed in later chapters, what can you do in your daily life to minimize the virus's progression?

Many scientists believe that since the virus lives within the immune system, any activation of that system has the potential to activate the virus. Some doctors and many HIV educators, I among them, encourage HIV+s to respond quickly to any health problems. This means:

- if you have a cold, rest;
- if you cut yourself, clean and treat the wound with antibiotics regularly;
- take care of all health problems as they arise;
- try to avoid concurrent infections.

I would not recommend that you take antibiotics for every infection, but if your doctor feels it is necessary, use antibiotics to help fight the infection and take the strain off your immune system. The point is, if your immune system is overactivated, the potential exists to activate the virus, since it lives in the immune system's cells.

With regard to this last point, remember: the information I give you is to help you reduce risk, not to increase worry. Actions you can take to avoid infections can be as simple as washing your hands more often. For a comprehensive review of simple infection-control procedures, see Chapter 16, Infection Control.

COFACTORS

Cofactors are conditions that put stress on the immune system, and in that way threaten to activate the virus in HIV+ people. In Chapter 2, I promised to stay with the known and wait for the facts to come in on cofactors. Here I want to clarify what I mean by that and help you sort through the debate so you can recognize the difference between *possible* and *actual* cofactors.

There's been a lot of dancing around the point when it comes to certain subjects. Let me say the words straight out:

- drugs
- alcohol
- cigarettes

All three are *known* cofactors that can speed up progression in HIV+ people.

RECREATIONAL DRUGS AND ALCOHOL

Let's start with drugs. I work on a daily basis with HIV+ recovering addicts in a residential treatment program. Whenever I see a patient who has just come back from using drugs for a couple of days, weeks, or months, blood is drawn to measure the immune system's strength and the measurements have usually dropped significantly.

These numbers are very difficult to rebuild—*almost impossible if the person continues to use drugs.* Laboratory tests have shown why. In a test tube, HIV replicates approximately 20 times faster in a solution containing cocaine than it does in a cocaine-free environment. With alcohol, the rate of replication is 5 times the control rate. Replication rates in other drug environments have not been tested, but I am convinced from personal observation that recreational drugs are dangerous for HIV+s.

John, a client who came to me eighteen months ago, had MAI, a serious AIDS-related infection (discussed in detail in Chapter 4; see Table 4-4). At the time, there were no FDA-approved drugs for MAI, but I knew of a medication called clarithromycin that was extremely effective in controlling this infection. The medication was available in Europe, and people in the United States could get it through buyers clubs (see page 147).

When I first met John, his doctor had given him two weeks to live. I personally went to the buyers club to purchase clarithromycin for John. I took the drug to him and he recovered completely and remained healthy for one year. Then he started to use recreational drugs again. As everyone knows, your priorities shift when you use drugs, and getting the medication to stay alive became secondary to John. He died within eight months.

I was furious with him, because I had fought the doctors and people at my job and had personally done the legwork to help him save his life—and he had killed himself. To this day, the story makes me very sad.

If you are on drugs, you don't have to be. There is help and hope. Alcoholics Anonymous and Narcotics Anonymous are great programs that work. Look in the yellow pages and get help. You don't have to die of HIV, and you certainly don't have to die of drug use.

There's a postscript to John's story: clarithromycin was later approved by the FDA and is currently available. Never give up hope. It's impossible to predict what's going to happen.

SMOKING

My suggestion about smoking is that you do the best you can to quit, but approach one thing at a time. If you are getting off drugs or alcohol, then wait until you are stable before you try to quit smoking. And if you have problems quitting, keep trying and give yourself credit for the attempt. The most important thing of all is not to add more stress to your life by beating yourself up.

Two studies reported at the Eighth International AIDS Conference in Amsterdam (PoB 3362 and PoB 3172) concluded that smoking increased the risk of developing HIV- and AIDS-related infections. Personally, I know one patient whose T4 cells rose by 200 within two months of giving up cigarettes, and I have collected many more stories of people feeling and getting better after quitting. There are other reports of smoking activating T4 cells, which can potentially activate the HIV virus. In the December 1992 issue of GMHC's *Treatment Issues,* smoking was also linked to impaired ability of wounds to heal and increased risk for developing precancerous abnormalities.

It just doesn't seem to be a good idea, in any sense. Try not to look at it as taking something away (the cigarettes) but as giving yourself a gift—the gift of health.

STRESS

Most lists of cofactors start with stress as the number-one problem. The significance of stress as a factor in HIV progression cannot be minimized. One study, conducted by Dr. Mary Anne Fletcher, director of the clinical immunology lab at the University of Miami, showed that T4-cell increases in people who reduced their stress levels equaled T4-cell increases in people on AZT during the same period of time. Think about when you are more likely to get a cold—is it when you are resting on a vacation or when you stay up late every night to complete a project? Trying to eliminate stress from your life makes sense, but not to the point of becoming crazy about it.

There's also such a thing as *positive* stress. Anything that results in an increase in self-esteem falls into that category. For example, a good relationship might be stressful, but in a positive, enriching, and exciting way. Psychotherapy can be stressful, but in a productive, insight-bringing way. And a challenging work project can be stressful, but in a way that galvanizes your energy and brings your talents and abilities into action.

There are many effective techniques for eliminating negative, energy-sapping stresses and anxieties. The easiest to use is *affirmation.* When your mind is running on and on, telling you that you have to do this and that, replace that chatter with another, more self-affirming thought—for example:

The chattering voice in your mind says, "I've *got* to take it easy, I'm supposed to be anxiety-free, if I don't relax I know I'm going to get sick, why can't I just quit running around and relax." The affirmation that replaces that message says, "I'm perfectly healthy, my T4 cells are rising and rising, I love myself just the way I am . . . *I am safe!*"

Stress is usually fear, so if you do a "reality check" to remind yourself that you are safe, you can usually reduce the pressure. A reality check is simply figuring out what's really happening *right now:*

- How important is the thing I'm worrying about?
- Will I get fired if I don't get it taken care of?
- Will I die if I don't?

Someone I know put it succinctly: "If it must get done, it *will* get done." That simple statement says it all.

Meditation is another great technique for reducing stress. You don't need anything fancy from another culture or another language. Just start your day with a five-minute period when you sit and listen to a quiet song in your mind and picture yourself in peaceful surroundings you love. For instance, if you love the beach, imagine you are there. This is a beautiful beach, with just the right air and water temperature for you, and the sun shining lightly on you while healing your body.

For more stress-reduction techniques, see Chapter 17, The Mind–Body Connection: Psychoneuroimmunology.

REINFECTION

The last cofactor I want to mention is reinfection. In Chapter 2, I explained the dangers of reinfection and increasing the viral load in your body, but I want to reiterate here that anyone with HIV does not need to add a different strain or type of the HIV virus to his or her system. I had one client who was in remission from HIV-related lymphoma and doing wonderfully. Her T4 cells had gone up to 550. But she had several unsafe sexual experiences with her HIV+ boyfriend, and within a month her T cells were at 149. Now, I don't know for certain whether the drop in the cell count was related to reinfection, but that was the only factor in her life at that time that had changed.

Let me tell you what I told her: Safer sex doesn't have to be a limitation. Not only does it give you the exquisite relief of knowing you are safe from reinfection, it can really be fun. But don't take my word for it. Experiment, explore, *play*!

Life's not over with an HIV diagnosis. A new phase of life has just begun.

BREAKING THE MYTHS

Myth: You can't live, at least not well, with a compromised immune system.
Truth: People all over the world are living well and are symptom-free, despite the facts that they test positive for the presence of HIV antibodies and their immune systems are severely compromised.

Myth: A negative antibody test always means you aren't infected.
Truth: In the window period, the antibody test comes up negative because the immune system hasn't yet produced antibodies in response to HIV infection. In fact, the viral load can be greatest before antibody production, and the blood can still test negative on the antibody test.

Myth: You can't get HIV-infected blood from a blood bank anymore.

Truth: You can be infected if the blood in a transfusion was drawn from an infected person before antibodies were produced.

Myth: Life is over with a positive diagnosis of HIV.
Truth: You're here, you're still you, and a *new* life is just beginning.

CHAPTER 4

HIV Evolution and Symptoms: An Overview

When I was drafting this chapter, I learned that two more of my patients had significant rises in T4 cells. I tell you this to reiterate that not everyone infected with the virus gets HIV-related infections and symptoms. One patient increased from 500 to 1,000; another from 120 to 550. This kind of positive change in blood values is a mystery to many doctors, but not to me. The information for achieving it is contained in this book, and it's relatively simple to apply.

As I go over the symptoms and conditions related to HIV infection and AIDS, we all need to remind ourselves that we are healthy and *living with HIV*. The information in this chapter is intended to empower you. If you tend to overidentify, you might want to read the chapter and tables—which list infections in detail—separately. (Tables 4-1, 4-2, and 4-4 appear at the end of the chapter.)

I keep interjecting favorable case histories to refute the ridiculous notion that HIV is an unconquerable monster that eats up everything it touches. True, living with and controlling the infection is a task that takes constant attention and monitoring, but it's far from impossible. People are surviving all around us. We can't count on the morning newspaper to spread these stories, so I'm taking every chance I can to do it here. Hearing or reading two or three survivors' stories over breakfast ought to be part of every prescribed treatment regimen, it can do that much good.

HIV infection is not AIDS, and in many cases does not necessarily involve symptoms at all. But if HIV infection is not an illness per se, what is it? Figure 4-1 answers this question best. It is a graphic representation of the spectrum of HIV infection showing that HIV infection is a *range* of conditions, from asymptomatic to AIDS.

Bear in mind one point above all as you familiarize yourself with this figure. The course of infection can go both ways across the symptom boundary—*toward* symptoms and *away* from them.

As far as we know, progression can and does stop at any point along the way. Your laboratory bloodwork, discussed in detail in the next chapter, is used to track the course of infection along this spectrum.

Infection and Dormancy

In some people the virus remains inactive or dormant. In some people, the virus has remained dormant for as long as we have known about it and have been tracking it. There are cases where we have tracked dormancy for eleven years, and counting.

The Window Period

Between infection and seroconversion is the "window period," during which the infected person can transmit the virus without knowing it. For instance, as a blood donor, this person would give infected blood, but in an antibody test this blood would register

FIGURE 4-1   The spectrum of HIV infection

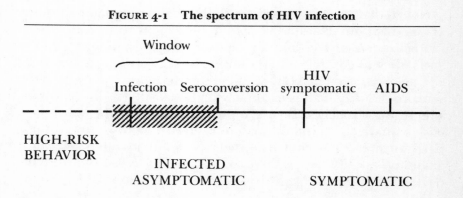

negative for the HIV virus. Furthermore, this person could be completely asymptomatic—that is, symptom-free.

How long does the window period last? Unfortunately, there is no definite answer to that question. Most people will make antibodies within six months, others within a year. But there are continual debates within the scientific community, and most believe there are a small number of cases in which it may take more than a year to produce antibodies.

Theoretically, the higher the concentrations of virus that enter the body—that is, the greater the viral load—the more quickly the body produces antibodies. This means that sexually transmitted HIV probably takes longer to show up on the antibody test than HIV transmitted by sharing needles, because more virus gets transmitted intravenously than sexually.

Seroconversion: Antibody Production

When you produce antibodies to HIV, you test positive on the HIV-antibody test. The change from negative to positive is called *seroconversion*.

After seroconversion, the infected person

- can infect another person
- will come up positive for HIV antibodies and would be considered HIV+ in a blood test
- immediately before seroconversion, or quite possibly during the process, develops a resistant flu that can be serious enough for the person to be hospitalized, and then finally resolves

Notice that seroconversion is still in the asymptomatic section of the diagram. The flu-like symptoms are probably caused by the activation of the immune system and its manufacture of antibodies to control the HIV virus. At this point, the body is effectively controlling HIV. Studies show that right *before* seroconversion, the viral load is extremely high—as high as in someone who is experiencing serious symptoms—but right afterward the body's unaffected immune system is able to gain control of the virus, bringing the viral load down to an almost undetectable amount.

HIV Asymptomatic

Once the body develops antibodies to the virus and the resistant flu disappears, the person usually enters a long period in which he or she is HIV+ but completely healthy—no symptoms, no nothing! This is a general statement, true for the most part but not in all cases. As I've said before, HIV manifests differently in each person, but there are similarities. For instance, some infected people can remain asymptomatic for ten years or more without medical intervention. Others get sick earlier. And some, to date, *have not gotten sick at all.* Up to this point, of the people who have been infected for ten years or more, 35 percent have not developed any serious HIV-related infection. HIV+ people in whom antibodies have been produced and who have no symptoms of HIV infection are called *HIV asymptomatic.*

HIV Symptomatic

The next step on the spectrum, symptomatic, is marked by the appearance of symptoms. To repeat (this fact is nearly universally overlooked by the popular media), there is no set time period between seroconversion and the onset of symptoms, and there is still a chance that some HIV+s will never progress. In addition, there is little information on HIV progression when medical and alternative treatments have been used.

My personal experience with patients is that with natural interventions (discussed in Chapter 8) early on, T4 cells rise and can stay above 1,000 for years. One of my patients, Steve, has maintained a T4-cell count of 600 and has been symptom-free since he found out he was HIV+ six years ago.

The point is, although the diagram is linear, there is no definite, clearly predictable pattern of progression in HIV infection.

WHAT'S IN A NAME? PLENTY!

The stage at which symptoms first show themselves was once commonly known as ARC, or AIDS-related complex. It is the Centers for Disease Control and Prevention (the CDC), a federal agency, which develops the names and diagnostic procedures for new diseases—in this case, ARC and AIDS. When HIV first appeared, the main concern, and still the driving force behind such decisions, was how to decide if a person would be eligible for benefits, which benefits the person would receive, and when the federal government would be exempt from paying health and support benefits.

In 1979, when the CDC first began researching HIV infection, its researchers began to see commonalities among clusters of immune-deficient people, whose condition was as yet unnamed. The agency compiled a list of "opportunistic infections" (OIs)— infections for which a compromised immune system offered an "opportunity" to develop. Unfortunately for many HIV-symptomatic people, the CDC decided that some of those OIs were less serious than others—a step that caused an unbelievable amount of grief and outrage, since people were dying of those "less serious" manifestations of HIV, just as they were from the "more serious" ones. Women, who were dying from these symptoms in disproportionate numbers, were not accounted for in the research. For a detailed description of the term *ARC,* which the CDC no longer uses, see page 59.

As you can see, the description of ARC was similar to a Chinese menu. For a diagnosis of ARC, you needed two symptoms from column A, or one from A and two from B, plus one or more from C, and at least two from D.

Confused yet?

Up until 1989, the government used these criteria for an ARC diagnosis to determine who would receive social security and Medicaid benefits—those who met the criteria for ARC and AIDS also qualified for benefits. But the federal government was soon alarmed to discover that people could live a very long time with ARC, maybe even forever—and the government could wind up supporting people for years and years. So they canceled the definition of ARC and now use the term *HIV symptomatic.* (Many doctors still use *ARC,* but the term is no longer recognized by the government.)

And HIV-symptomatic people are *not* entitled to federal benefits.

Do people die of HIV-related symptoms?

Yes, especially women, who were not even included in the original research in which the definitions were developed.

The CDC's Definition of ARC

Clinical
Requirements: two major findings (column A)
AND immunological (one or more from column C)
AND other lab (two or more from column D)

or

one major finding (column A)
AND two or more minor findings (column B)
AND immunological (one or more from column C)
AND other lab (two or more from column D)

Column A	Column B
Clinical Major	Clinical Minor
Lymphadenopathy	Night sweats ≥ 3 months
Thrush in the mouth	Fatigue
Hairy leukoplakia	Pruritis (itching) ≥ 1 month
Herpes zoster (shingles)	Extensive seborrheic
Fever ≥ 3 months	Dermatitis or eczema
Central or peripheral neurologic	Refractory dermatophytosis
deficit	(skin fungus)
Diarrhea ≥ 3 months	Contagiosum blisters (skin
	infection)
	Unexplained sinusitis

Column C
Immunological

Helper T-cell count under 400/cubic mm
Helper/suppressor ratio ≤ 1.0
Cutaneous anergy (negative to 3 or more skin test. Lack of response
to antigens)

Column D
Other Laboratory

Leukopenia: abnormal decrease of white blood cells ≤ 400 cubic mm
Lymphopenia: deficiency of lymphocytes ≤ 1,000 cubic mm
Anemia: hematocrit ≤ 35
Thrombocytopenia: abnormal decrease in number of blood platelets
Lowered serum cholesterol ≤ 135 mg
Sedimentation rate ≥ 20
HIV antibody or virus culture positive

THE SYMPTOMS OF HIV INFECTION

Table 4-1, HIV-Related Infections, covers infections, symptoms, specific causes, and diagnostic procedures of HIV-related infections. Other issues—such as prevention and treatment—will be covered in later chapters.

On the table, which lists infections in alphabetical order, I've included:

- the name of the infection plus any alternative medical names and any "street" names
- the cause, which covers the type of transmission agent—protozoan, virus, fungi—and how it is spread
- the diagnostic procedure—how the condition is diagnosed—both *presumptive* (if the condition looks like it and responds to the usual treatment for it, then it's it) and *definitive* (usually through biopsy or other invasive procedures to ascertain the agent and culture in a lab)
- the common symptoms
- any other facts you should know

Table 4-2, HIV-Related Symptoms in Women, rights the terrible imbalance that has excluded women from many descriptions of symptoms—and therefore, all too often, from receiving accurate diagnosis and treatment. It covers HIV-related symptoms, listed in alphabetical order, that affect women *only*. But please note: women can get the conditions described on both tables, so if you are a woman you should acquaint yourself with *all* the symptom information on *both* tables, not just that on Table 4-2. For a fuller discussion of those issues affecting women exclusively, see Chapter 11, Special Concerns of Women.

While it's important to describe these infections thoroughly, I want to avoid creating hypochondriacal HIV+ readers. The symptoms listed on the table affect many people but not everyone. Some people don't get sick at all, even when their bloodwork has changed significantly. Others, with intervention, do not even have blood-value deficiencies. So try to read about these symptoms in a neutral way, receiving the information without—as far as it is possible—letting it trigger your imagination.

WHAT IS AIDS?

At the beginning of the 1980s, the CDC, as the central reporting agency, began getting word of a new illness among gay men that some were calling GRID (Gay-Related Immune Deficiency). As the agency worked on developing a way for doctors to diagnose this condition, CDC personnel began to notice that similar symptoms were surfacing among addicts who were not necessarily gay. They knew, therefore, that the illness was not, as they had first believed, restricted to the gay community.

As more and more data was collected, it became clear that this condition qualified as a *syndrome*, a condition that causes several other diseases or symptoms. Accordingly, the CDC named it acquired immunodeficiency syndrome, or AIDS.

In refining its guidelines on AIDS diagnosis, the CDC gathered research and compared people with similar infections. From these, they chose the "most serious" infections—infections they predicted would result in an eighteen-month to three-year life span after first appearing—and made these the criteria for the diagnosis of AIDS. The agency's final list consisted of the "opportunistic infections" (OIs) listed (in alphabetical order) in Table 4-3. Any person who is diagnosed with one of the infections on this list is diagnosed with AIDS as well. Some of these OIs are more commonly known by the names or abbreviations in parentheses.

When the list was first compiled, an understanding of the HIV virus and testing procedures were not yet in place. Today, to be diagnosed with AIDS, you must be HIV+ in addition to having one of the conditions on the list.

Excellent treatments now exist for many of the listed infections that were not treatable then. In addition, some of the infections—for example, Kaposi's sarcoma, or KS—turned out to be not as "serious" as the CDC thought they were, and people were living with them much longer than was expected. For those reasons, the CDC has tried—unsuccessfully—to eliminate some of the infections from the list.

Meanwhile, it became clear to people outside the CDC that the list wasn't comprehensive *enough*. Owing to the many "actions" launched by activists to pressure the agency, the CDC planned to expand the definition of AIDS in January of 1992, but no

TABLE 4-3

The CDC List of AIDS-Diagnosing OIs (In Alphabetical Order)

1. Candidiasis, bronchi, trachea, lungs (thrush)
2. Candidiasis, esophageal (thrush)
3. Coccidiomycosis, disseminated or extrapulmonary
4. Cryptococcosis, extrapulmonary (crypto)
5. Cryptosporidiosis, chronic intestinal
6. Cytomegalovirus disease (CMV)
7. Cytomegalovirus retinitis (CMV/eyes)
8. HIV encephalopathy (dementia)
9. Herpes simplex, chronic ulcers (HSV)
10. Histoplasmosis (histo)
11. Isosporiasis, chronic intestinal
12. Kaposi's sarcoma (KS)
13. Lymphoma, Burkitt's
14. Lymphoma, immunoblastic
15. Lymphoma, primary in brain
16. *Mycobacterium avium* complex or M. kansasii (MAC)
17. *M. tuberculosis,* disseminated or extrapulmonary (TB)
18. Mycobacterium of other species
19. *Pneumocystis carinii* pneumonia (PCP)
20. Progressive multifocal leukoencephalopathy (PML)
21. Salmonella septicemia, recurrent
22. Toxoplasmosis of brain (toxo)
23. Wasting syndrome

The CDC added the following to its list on January 1, 1993:
24. *M. tuberculosis,* pulmonary (TB)
25. Recurrent pneumonias within a 12-month period
26. Invasive cervical cancer
27. T_4 (CD_4) cells under 200, or less than 14 percent

changes were made. However, as of January 1, 1993, the CDC officially added the following four criteria to its list defining AIDS:

- T4 cells below 200 or less than 14 percent (applicable to adolescents and adults)
- pulmonary tuberculosis (*extrapulmonary* tuberculosis, or tuberculosis outside the lungs, was on the original list)
- recurrent pneumonias within a twelve-month period
- invasive cervical cancer

The latter item was the CDC's concession to pressure to include conditions specific to women, which had been overlooked before. When the agency first compiled its list, it failed to take women into account at all and did not recognize particular infections as manifestations of the syndrome in females.

It is good to stay informed. The AIDS Hot Line (listed in the Resource Guide, Chapter 20) can confirm the most recent criteria.

Again, as with ARC, the whole idea of this list was solely intended to determine who would receive government benefits! Though the list remains nearly unchanged, however, it's important to remember that new treatments and alternatives are extending lives. People live five, eight, ten years, and counting. Only God knows how many days you have left. No doctor can ever tell you that and be certain.

The most alarming thing about these lists is that they cause people emotional distress. Take, for example, the new criterion of a T4 count below 200. This is one of those categories in which people are alive for ten years *plus*. But whenever I'm in a group and mention that now everyone with a T4-cell count below 200 will be diagnosed with AIDS, I can see the faces become grim. People ask, "Does that mean I have AIDS? I've never been sick, but I have 180 T4 cells."

Don't read more meaning into this criterion than there is. If your T4-cell count is below 200, this only means that you are now eligible for benefits. You're no sicker than you were yesterday!

Table 4-4, AIDS-Diagnosing OIs, describes many AIDS-related infections (in alphabetical order), providing symptoms and related information.

Remember, AIDS is just a four-letter word.

BREAKING THE MYTHS

Myth: Everyone with HIV will get sick.

Truth: Although many doctors and scientists are theorizing that this is true, it is not a confirmed fact. Thirteen years after becoming infected, 35 percent of the HIV+ people tracked in the San Francisco Clinic Cohort study, a report by Dr. Susan Buchbinder, et al., have not developed AIDS. Of that 35 percent, 25 percent have fewer than 200 T4 cells, 50 percent have between 200 and 500 T4s, and the remaining 25 percent have T4-cell counts in the normal range, above 500.

All the facts are not in yet. It is still possible that some HIV+s

(*continued on page 84*)

TABLE 4-1   **HIV-Related Infections**

Condition	Cause (Agent of Transmission)	Diagnostic Procedure
Diarrhea	Can be a parasite. Anal oral sex (rimming) can transmit diarrhea-causing agents. In addition, the source of diarrhea can be an OI (MAI/MAC [see Table 4-4] can cause diarrhea) or HIV virus itself.	Self-report of diarrhea Complete workup Stool testing
Fevers	Unknown	Thermometer
Fungal infections	Fungi Usually transmitted on towels, hands, washcloths, sheets, bathroom mats Contagious	Definitive: usually visual exam
Generalized or persistent lymphadenopathy	Unknown	Medical exam. Lymphoma should be ruled out.
Hairy leukoplakia	Unknown viral agent associated with forms of the herpes virus, specifically Epstein-Barr virus (EBV) and human papillomavirus (HPV) Noncontagious	Visual exam
Herpes zoster (shingles)	Varicella-zoster virus (VZV), the chickenpox virus. In people previously infected with chickenpox, latent VZV resides in the nerve roots. When it is reactivated, shingles occurs.	Presumptive: visual exam Definitive: culture of lesion or tissue biopsy

TABLE 4-1   **HIV-Related Infections (continued)**

Symptoms	*Comments*
Persistent watery bowel	Whether you test positive for parasites or not, treat with the herbal preparation described in Chapter 8. This treatment is simple and totally nontoxic. Parasites can hide in stool samples and false negative readings are common. Check for MAI and cryptosporidiosis when T4 cells are below 100 or 5 percent (see Table 4-4).
Persistent low-grade fevers	Have a complete workup. Check for MAI when T4 cells are below 100 or 5 percent (see Table 4-4).
Discolored toenails, fingernails, patches of discolored or red skin, itching, dry, cracking between toes, flaking skin	Avoid sharing towels. If infected, use separate towels for the infected area and use only once before laundering.
Swollen lymph nodes (often called swollen glands) under arms, in neck, groin, etc. Generalized lymphadenopathy may affect any lymph node. May be accompanied by fevers	Most health-care professionals consider swollen glands a sign that the immune system is working; therefore, this is a symptom of a positive nature. The condition is usually persistent, can be uncomfortable, and is visually unappealing. This condition does not represent progressive disease and usually causes no problems.
White patches in the mouth, usually on the tongue	Can be confused with thrush, which has a similar appearance in the mouth. However, thrush can usually be brushed off the tongue, while hairy leukoplakia cannot. The patches are white and feel leathery within the mouth. Make sure the diagnosis is certain—the treatments for thrush and hairy leukoplakia are very different.
Blistery, painful lesions that form a cluster	Herpes zoster usually affects the face and trunk on one side of the body. The lesions follow the paths of sensory nerves, so you can see a definite line where they stop. Rarely are the lesions disseminated (meaning they can be anywhere on the body).

Table 4-1	HIV-Related Infections (continued)	
Condition	Cause (Agent of Transmission)	Diagnostic Procedure
Herpes zoster (shingles) (continued)	Can be contagious if you are exposed to oozing sores. Before blisters burst or once they heal, noncontagious.	
HPV (human papillomavirus), genital warts	Virus transmitted through sexual contact.	Presumptive: visual exam
	Contagious but usually prevented by condom use	Definitive: Pap smears, biopsy
Idiopathic thrombocytopenia purpura (ITP) (HIV-related low-platelet count)	Unknown. Somehow the body produces antibodies that attack the blood platelets, the cells that cause the blood to clot.	Definitive: simple platelet-count blood test
	Definitely more common in HIV+s	
	Completely noncontagious	
Mouth and dental problems	Unknown. Immune suppression probably causes exposure to everyday bacteria to produce symptoms. Usually routine in people with healthy immune systems; serious in the immunosuppressed	Dental exam
Night sweats	Unknown	Self-report
Neuropathy (peripheral neuropathy)	HIV itself seems to cause this condition. It can be the result of drug toxicities; ddC and ddI commonly cause this condition	Self-report
	Noncontagious	

TABLE 4-1   **HIV-Related Infections (continued)**

Symptoms	*Comments*
Warts in genital area, including vagina, vulva, cervix, penis, outer anus, and anal canal	Extremely common in HIV+ women. See Table 4-2.
Excessive bleeding from nosebleeds, injuries, or cuts. Some people bruise easily. Small and large red spots on skin	No need to look for symptoms—any decent health-care professional should be doing regular platelet counts and should diagnose ITP early. It is important to treat this disorder early. Common treatment is prednisone, a steroid that shuts down the immune system. This is *totally unacceptable*, since gamma globulin, a nontoxic immune modulator, can be just as effective. See the treatment table for additional information.
Pain in mouth. Sores can be herpetic and are easily treated	Prevention with good oral hygiene; regular and proper exams.
Waking in drenched clothes and sheets. Literally soaking or wringing wet sheets can be common	Have a complete workup. Check for MAI when T4 cells are below 100 or 5 percent (see Table 4-4).
Pain, tingling, numbness in feet and legs, sometimes hands and fingers. Pain may be severe and walking difficult	Neuropathy may be a side effect of a current treatment; if so, you need to measure benefit against toxicity. Peptide T, now being tested in drug trials, is available through buyers clubs. It is currently the best treatment for neuropathy.

TABLE 4-1   HIV-Related Infections (continued)

Condition	Cause (Agent of Transmission)	Diagnostic Procedure
Nonspecific dermatitis (skin disorders)— seborrhea, psoriasis, pruritis (itching)	Unknown Noncontagious	Definitive: usually visual exam
Recurrent bacterial infections	Bacterial agents common to HIV+s cause pneumonias, flus, strep throat. Most of these bacteria are present in air, blood, water, and the human body. Contagious	Sometimes difficult to pin down specific agent. Suggest treating presumptively
Sinusitis	Unknown	Self-report
Syphilis (latent and recurrent)	Bacterium. Sexually transmitted. Prevent by condom use	Blood test, titer level. (When the term *titer* is used, the measurement usually reflects the level or amount of infection—the higher the range, the more dangerous and/or active the infection.)
Thrush (candida, or candidiasis)	A yeastlike fungus (*Candida albicans* is the most common) that is present in all people but that grows out of control when the immune system is compromised Noncontagious	Presumptive: visual exam Definitive: culture or smear

TABLE 4-1   **HIV-Related Infections (continued)**

Symptoms	Comments
Itching, blotches, red rashes, dandruff, scabbing	Early, aggressive intervention is recommended.
Fevers, night sweats, swollen glands, productive cough, shortness of breath	Vaccines, i.e., pneumovax vaccine, can prevent many of these infections.
Watery, persistent sinus condition; difficulty breathing	Check for allergies. See if allergy shots are feasible.
In primary syphilis there may be no symptoms at all—that's why a titer test is a must Chancre sores or lesions are the most common early symptoms. See Table 4-2 for more symptoms	Most common in HIV+ women. See Table 4-2 for details.
A white coating in the mouth. (See Table 4-2 for vaginal thrush or yeast infections.) In any HIV+ person, yeast can grow out of control in other areas, such as the large intestine or lungs	Thrush in the mouth or vagina or on the skin is HIV symptomatic. Thrush in the bronchi, trachea, esophagus, or lungs is the basis for an AIDS diagnosis. These arbitrary distinctions are sometimes confusing, but we must keep in mind that money is the deciding factor. When people have thrush in the throat they cannot eat, so the condition is supposedly more life-threatening than when it affects other sites. That explains the AIDS diagnosis: the government believes that people with thrush in the throat will get financial benefits but will not live too long. On the other hand, so the thinking goes, with thrush in the mouth or vagina, people can live forever. The problem with this distinction is that thrush is easily treated and people can live forever *whatever the site*.

TABLE 4-2   **HIV-Related Symptoms in Women**

Condition	Cause (Agent of Transmission)	Diagnostic Procedure
Abnormal Pap smears; cervical cancers	Nontransmissible	When Pap smear is abnormal, follow with colposcopy.
Chlamydia	Sexually transmitted disease	Most accurate test is culture
Chronic vaginitis or vaginal yeast infections (vaginal thrush)	With yeast: fungus; grows out of control when immune system is compromised Can also be trichomonal vaginitis, caused by a parasite, and is transmitted sexually	Presumptive: GYN exam Definitive: culture or smear (smear is more common and more conclusive)
Herpes (genital)	Virus Sexually transmitted	Presumptive: visual exam Definitive: viral culture
Neoplasia ("new growth")—cervical interstitial neoplasia; lower-tract neoplasia	Early cancer condition; nontransmissible	Pap smear
Penicillin-resistant gonorrhea (PPNG)	Sexually transmitted disease	Make sure lab culture is tested for PPNG as well as regular gonorrhea
PID (pelvic inflammatory disease)	Untreated sexually transmitted diseases can progress, causing pelvic abscess. Chlamydia is a common STD that causes PID.	Regular GYN exams for PPNG, chlamydia, gonorrhea, HPV, Pap smears, and syphilis

TABLE 4-2   HIV-Related Symptoms in Women (continued)

Symptoms	Comments
None	The earlier the diagnosis, the more successful the treatment. Have regular colposcopy.
Women usually remain symptom-free while underlying pelvic damage occurs. In some but not all cases, vaginal discharge can be present. If left untreated, pain, fever, miscarriage, and infertility can occur.	Avoid complications by testing regularly during exams. There is a long asymptomatic phase, so multiple testing in GYN exams is strongly advised.
Burning, itching, white discharge, coating, distinctive odor, redness, pain during intercourse	Extremely common in HIV+ women. Dietary adjustment immensely beneficial; avoid bread (yeast), alcohol, dairy foods, and sugar.
Lesions, may be internal; careful GYN exam recommended	Herpes is a definite cofactor in the activation of HIV infection. Diagnosis and preventative treatments are recommended.
None	Easily treated with early diagnosis
Burning when urinating; discharge	Penicillin-resistant but treatable. This is another infection that can remain undetected, putting undue stress on the immune system. Treat aggressively and eliminate.
Vaginal discharge, pain, internal abscesses, ectopic pregnancy, constitutional symptoms	Ectopic pregnancy is a major cause of maternal mortality. Regular GYN exams and the close following of the recommendations on this table can, in most cases, prevent PID.

TABLE 4-2　HIV-Related Symptoms in Women (continued)

Condition	Cause (Agent of Transmission)	Diagnostic Procedure
Syphilis (latent or recurrent)	Spirochetal bacterium (*Treponema pallidum*). This is a sexually transmitted disease and can be prevented with a condom.	Blood test; measurement of titer. False negatives are common. Test regularly and have health-care worker use different types of syphilis tests to be sure you are infection-free. A spinal tap is often necessary.
Vaginal warts (human papillomavirus, HPV)	Virus; sexually transmitted	Presumptive: GYN exam Definitive: culture, Pap smears (both cervical and anal)

TABLE 4-2   HIV-Related Symptoms in Women (continued)

Symptoms	Comments
Primary syphilis can often be symptom-free except for a chancre sore at the site of infection which may disappear resulting in a long asymptomatic period. Symptoms for secondary syphilis can include rash, lymphadenopathy (swollen nodes, also common in general HIV infection), fevers, diarrhea, and other constitutional symptoms. Latent syphilis can affect organs.	Treat aggressively. Often, hospitalization for intravenous antibiotic is treatment of choice. Check titer regularly, since syphilis can recur and titer can rise. Aggressive intravenous antibiotic treatment is the most successful.
Warts can be seen and felt if external; if internal requires examination	Women with HPV must have regular Pap smears, since HPV has been linked with cervical cancer. HPV can be recurrent, so follow-up after treatment is essential. HIV does not always cause vaginal warts, so culture is important even if there are no symptoms. In one study, 26 percent of HIV-infected women had HPV.

TABLE 4-4   AIDS-Diagnosing OIs

Condition	Cause/Agent/ Mode of Transmission	Diagnostic Procedure
Candidiasis (thrush) (AIDS diagnosing only when affecting the esophagus, bronchi, trachea, or lungs)	*Candida albicans*, a yeastlike fungus. As the immune system becomes compromised, the yeast, which is present in all people, grows out of control. Noncontagious	Presumptive: mouth—visual exam vagina—GYN exam esophagus—recent onset of pain behind the sternum during swallowing and visual exam Definitive: microscopic exam of sputum obtained directly from affected tissues
Coccidiomycosis, disseminated or extrapulmonary	A fungus (*Coccidioides immitis*)	Definitive: Microscopic exam of sputum or specimen obtained with a bronchioscope
Cryptococcosis, extrapulmonary (cryptococcal meningitis)	*Cryptococcus neoformans*, a fungus	Definitive: microscopic exam of cells or tissue culture, or detection of an antigen in a specimen or from affected tissues or fluid (such as cerebrospinal fluid) For pneumonia—chest X ray With neurological symptoms—CAT scan or MRI to rule out other brain infections; spinal tap
Cryptosporidiosis, chronic intestinal	Infection is caused by a parasite, *Cryptosporidium*. Contagious; spread through oral contact with feces of an infected animal or oralanal contact (rimming) with an infected person	Stool tests (repeat tests are often required), bowel biopsy, endoscopy. Microscopic exam of cells or tissue

TABLE 4-4   **AIDS-Diagnosing OIs (continued)**

Symptoms	*Comments*
A quick-growing fungus appearing in the mouth, esophagus, lungs, bronchi, trachea, pharynx, oral and vaginal mucosa, skin, and gastrointestinal tract. Also appears as inflammation around the fingernails. Mouth: white coating in the mouth Vagina: burning, itching, white discharge and coating, odor, redness, pain during intercourse Esophagus: pain, difficulty swallowing	The fungus normally inhabits the body, causing no harm in people with healthy immune systems. In people with immune suppression, can appear wherever the skin or mucous membrane is damaged, including IV therapy and pressure-monitoring sites, and the like. Only an AIDS-diagnosing disease when it affects the esophagus, bronchi, trachea, or lungs. Can cause pain and wasting when it interferes with eating and swallowing. Thrush in the mouth or vagina is often an early sign of HIV infection and is not a basis for a diagnosis of AIDS.
Nonspecific symptoms: malaise, weight loss, fatigue, cough	Mostly infects the lungs, but in an advanced form the disease can affect the kidneys, spleen, lymph nodes, brain, and thyroid gland
Most commonly affects the brain. Also affects lungs and other organs. In lungs can cause a form of pneumonia mimicking or occurring with PCP. Mental confusion, intermittent low-grade fevers, progressive weakness, fatigue, headache, nausea, vomiting, meningeal signs (double vision; stiff neck), memory loss, altered mental state, seizures (rare)	The organism is a yeastlike fungus found worldwide, often in soil contaminated with bird excrement. It is usually acquired by inhalation.
Severe diarrhea with frequent watery stools, abdominal cramping, nausea, vomiting, flatulence, weight loss, loss of appetite, constipation, dehydration, electrolyte imbalances, malaise, fever	It is possible to be infected but be asymptomatic.

TABLE 4-4   **AIDS-Diagnosing OIs (continued)**

Condition	Cause/Agent/ Mode of Transmission	Diagnostic Procedure
Cytomegalovirus disease (CMV); cytomegalovirus retinitis	A herpes virus found in saliva, semen, cervical secretions, urine, feces, blood, and breast milk	For presence of virus: testing for CMV titer (levels) in the blood For retinitis Presumptive: Self-administered vision test (called "Amsler Grid") Definitive: eye exam For other types: biopsy, endoscopy, microscopic exam of cells or tissues
Herpes simplex, chronic ulcers	Virus (herpes simplex virus, HSV) Type 1 is spread by contact with infected oral secretions Type 2 is spread by contact with infected genital secretions Both types can be spread through touching lesions and then other body parts Contagious when a sore is present	Presumptive: visual exam Definitive: viral culture
Histoplasmosis	A fungus (*Histoplasma capulatum*)	Blood culture, bone-marrow biopsy and culture, lymph-node biopsy, or skin-lesion biopsy

TABLE 4-4   **AIDS-Diagnosing OIs (continued)**

Symptoms	*Comments*
General: fever, profound tiredness, muscle and joint aches, night sweats The virus causes different symptoms in different organs. retinitis (eyes): blurry eyesight leading to blindness; other vision problems include floating spots, loss of peripheral vision, and blind spots; resolution of active disease leaves scarring, mottling, and atrophying of the retina. esophagus (throat): pain, difficulty swallowing, ulceration colitis (colon): fever, diarrhea, abdominal pain, wasting pneumonia (rare); see PCP for symptoms liver: hepatitis	Infection by CMV is usually no problem in people with healthy immune systems. In people with compromised immune systems, the virus can cause active disease. Some terminology: In eyes—CMV retinitis In colon—CMV colitis In lungs—CMV pneumonia In brain—CMV encephalopathy This is one of the most commonly undiagnosed underlying conditions that is a cofactor in HIV progression. There is a study that already suggests CMV and other herpes viruses may be responsible for a significant amount of damage to the immune system well before these viruses are recognized or diagnosed. Some doctors are exploring ways to address herpes viruses with the hope that this might help stabilize and protect from future immune suppression. Recently, an oral trial of the CMV antiviral drug DHPG has been started to prophylax HIV+s with less than 100 T4 cells from serious CMV disease. It would not be surprising if other benefits from this prophylaxis become evident. Using Zovirax is recommended for prevention (see Chapter 14, Preventive Therapy).
Nonhealing blisters lasting more than one month on skin, especially around the anus, genitals, or mouth (nonmucous skin). Lesions are painful; can burn and itch. Sometimes: colitis, pericarditis, esophagitis, pneumonia. (HSV esophagitis appears with symptoms similar to CMV or candida.)	Lesions may be internal. In women, a careful GYN exam is recommended. Herpes is a definite cofactor in activating HIV infection. Diagnosis and preventive treatment recommended.
Fever, chills, muscle aches, headache, abdominal pain, weight loss, skin lesions, breathing difficulties, anemia, swollen lymph nodes	Can be difficult to diagnose

TABLE 4-4 AIDS-Diagnosing OIs (continued)		
Condition	Cause/Agent/ Mode of Transmission	Diagnostic Procedure
HIV encephalopathy (dementia, dementia complex, AIDS dementia syndrome)	HIV in the brain	Definitive: Diagnosed when conditions other than HIV encephalopathy have been ruled out by examining CSF and/ or by CAT or MRI of the brain.
Isosporiasis, chronic intestinal	A protozoan (*Isospora beill*) acquired from eating uncooked beef or pork or from an infected person through oral sexual contact	Fecal smear (antibody test unavailable)
Kaposi's sarcoma (KS)	A cancer whose cause is undetermined— possibly a contagious viral or bacterial sexually transmitted disease	Presumptive: visual exam (should be done by clinicians with significant experience with KS) Definitive: microscopic exam of cells or tissue; biopsy
Lymphomas: primary CNS lymphoma, systemic non-Hodgkin's lymphoma, and Hodgkin's disease	Lymphoma is sixty times more common in AIDS patients than in immune competent individuals.	Primary CNS lymphoma Presumptive: MRI and CAT scans; in some cases examination of the spinal fluid may provide diagnosis. Definitive: Brain biopsy (though rarely done owing to the complications of the procedure)

TABLE 4-4   AIDS-Diagnosing OIs (continued)

Symptoms	Comments
Neurological problems, from slight to severe—including decreased concentration, slowed thought, loss of interest, slowed motor movements. Balance, memory problems; slurred speech; personality changes. In children, loss of developmental milestones	HIV+ children are frequently affected. Although the condition results from HIV infection, the cause of the neurological symptoms remains unclear. Peptide T, still in trials, shows signs of resolving this condition.
Watery diarrhea (noninflammatory), abdominal pain and cramps, vomiting, anorexia, weight loss, fever, weakness. Indistinguishable from symptoms of cryptosporidiosis	Most commonly found in tropical and subtropical climates
Purple, reddish, or brown, usually nonsymmetrical lesions (nodules raised above skin) on external or internal organs, sometimes accompanied by edema. Lesions mostly involve the skin, but often involve lymph nodes, oral cavity, gastrointestinal tract, and lungs. Pulmonary involvement can cause severe respiratory symptoms.	Usually not life-threatening, KS is the most commonly diagnosed cancer in HIV-infected people. Before HIV, KS was seen only in North African and Southern European men in their seventies and eighties. There have been recent reports of successful treatment with the natural substance shark cartilade (see pages 164).
CNS: paralysis of one side of the body, loss of ability to speak or understand language, confusion, memory loss, seizures, apathy, lethargy; in some cases a headache is the only symptom	On MRI and CAT scans the lesions of primary lymphoma in the brain can be confused with those of toxoplasmosis of the brain. Both single and multiple lesions are seen. Primary lymphoma in the brain is usually a late complication of AIDS and difficult to treat.

TABLE 4-4   **AIDS-Diagnosing OIs (continued)**

Condition	Cause/Agent/ Mode of Transmission	Diagnostic Procedure
M. tuberculosis, disseminated or extrapulmonary (TB outside the lungs)	Mycobacterial infection: *Mycobacterium tuberculosis*. Contagious, but only during a two-week period and before treatments are begun	Definitive: sputum smear and culture (a PPD test, used to diagnose TB, is a skin test in which sensitivity is usually reduced in HIV+ people infected with TB, so these tests are unreliable), and blood, urine, lymph node, bone marrow, or other cultures
Mycobacterium avium complex (MAC) or *Mycobacterium* intracellular (MAI)	A mycobacterium found in soil, water, animals, eggs, unpasteurized dairy products, and other food. The infection is noncommunicable—it cannot be transmitted between people.	Presumptive: persistent high fevers, weight loss, and diarrhea with T4 cells below 70 Definitive: culture (though difficult to culture and not always found); should be treated presumptively in most cases
Pneumocystis carinii pneumonia (PCP)	Protozoan parasite	Presumptive: report of labored breathing when climbing stairs or with exertion over last three months, dry cough of recent onset, *no* evidence of bacterial pneumonia, and response to treatment Definitive: microscopic exam of sputum, chest X ray, gallium scan, bronchoscopy, blood-gas measurement, open-lung biopsy
Progressive multifocal leukoencephalopathy (PML)	Virus, JC virus	Presumptive: Abnormalities on brain MRI or CAT scan Definitive: microscopic exam of cells or tissues

TABLE 4-4 AIDS-Diagnosing OIs (continued)

Symptoms	*Comments*
Fever, cough, spitting up blood, night sweats, weight loss, fatigue, swollen lymph nodes. Note: in people with AIDS, these classic TB symptoms do not necessarily indicate TB. In lungs the symptoms resemble those of PCP.	In people with healthy immune systems, TB outside the lungs is rare, but among HIV+s at least half the TB cases involve sites outside the lungs. The central nervous system and lymphatic systems are often involved. In January 1993, pulmonary TB became the basis for an AIDS diagnosis, as well as the present extrapulmonary TB.
Persistent fever, weakness, night sweats, anorexia, weight loss, dizziness, nausea, abdominal pain, diarrhea, flu-like symptoms, shortness of breath, possible cough. Enlarged lymph nodes, frequently on one side, enlarged liver and spleen; soft-tissue masses (particularly in thighs)	In people with healthy immune systems, symptoms are usually limited to the respiratory system. Where the immune system is suppressed, infection can involve almost any organ system, but contamination is usually through the lungs or gastrointestinal tract. This condition may begin as a lung infection and then move (disseminate) to other organs, including the blood and bone marrow. Can also be spread throughout the system. Usually affects people with T4 cells below 70. This is a common underlying OI for which prophylaxis is important. The terms MAC and MAI are used interchangeably.
Dry cough, shortness of breath, difficulty breathing, fever, night sweats, weight loss, fatigue, chest pain, sputum production in late disease	This is the most commonly diagnosed AIDS OI. *P. carinii* is found in air, water, and soil, is carried by domestic animals and rodents, and may be latent in most people. Primary site of disease is lungs, but infection sometimes spreads to spleen, lymph nodes, and blood and, rarely, to the bone marrow and liver.
Memory loss, motor-control problems, seizures, mood changes, neurological symptoms and signs (e.g., weakness of one limb or one	Profound dementia can result from advanced disease.

TABLE 4-4   AIDS-Diagnosing OIs (continued)

Condition	Cause/Agent/ Mode of Transmission	Diagnostic Procedure
Pulmonary tuberculosis (TB in the lungs)	*Mycobacterium tuberculosis*. Before medication is begun, TB is contagious. The mycobacterium is present in sputum droplets, released into the air by coughing. Poor air circulation and not using masks can increase the chances of exposure. For non-HIV+ people, after exposure the chances of becoming actively ill are low. For HIV+s, the chances of active infection are much higher. Long-term exposure—e.g., via roommates—holds the greatest risk. Noncontagious several days after treatment begins	Reaction to PPD (purified protein derivative). Shallow injection of PPD will swell if exposed. Also, sputum tests (cultured for TB) and X rays. If immune compromised, PPD might give false negative. Use anergy panel to confirm results if T4s are below 500.
Salmonella septicemia, recurrent (Salmonellosis)	Bacteria. Infection results from ingestion of contaminated food and water. The bacteria multiply after entering the small intestine.	Bacterial culture of stool or blood
Toxoplasmosis of the brain	Protozoan (*Toxoplasma gondii*) passed by contact with infected cats and ingestion of raw or undercooked meat or unpasteurized dairy products. Mothers can transmit the organism to unborn children, but	Presumptive: Positive antibody test and CAT or MRI scan showing lesions Definitive: microscopic exam of tissues or cells; brain biopsy (rarely)

TABLE 4-4   **AIDS-Diagnosing OIs (continued)**

Symptoms	*Comments*
side of the body, loss of vision on one side, loss of feeling on one side or in one limb, language problems, unsteadiness)	
Cough, bloody sputum, shortness of breath, fever, weight loss, chest pain, fatigue, night sweats	In general, the PPD skin test must be done with another reaction-based skin test, the anergy panel, used as a control, since many people with HIV do not react to the PPD, even if they have been exposed to TB. If you react to the anergy panel, which is used to tell if your immune system is still mounting responses, you will probably react to the PPD. If the anergy panel is nonresponsive, a sputum and/or X ray is necessary.
Fever, chills, sweats, weight loss, diarrhea, anorexia	Although enterocolitis is common in people with AIDS, it is not usually caused by *salmonella*.
Produces lesions in the central nervous system, so symptoms are neurological: headaches, fever, chills, motor changes, lethargy, confusion, seizures, paralysis on one side of the body, delusions,	The organism accounts for the most widespread latent central-nervous-system infection in the world. The antibody test is not definitive.

TABLE 4-4 AIDS-Diagnosing OIs (continued)		
Condition	*Cause/Agent/ Mode of Transmission*	*Diagnostic Procedure*
	otherwise it cannot be transmitted between people.	
Wasting syndrome	Can vary—usually due to poor absorption. Tumor nucrosis factor (TNF) and glutathione levels have been linked to wasting syndrome.	Presumptive: Profound weight loss (more than 10 percent of baseline body weight) plus chronic diarrhea *or* weakness in the absence of other infections or conditions, and some-times accompanied by fevers

might never progress. And who knows what is going to happen to people who intervene very early with natural substances?

Myth: AIDS is a diagnosis originally created to denote a serious illness.
Truth: AIDS is a diagnosis used to determine who gets benefits.

Myth: Women get the same "opportunistic infections" as men.
Truth: Before January 1, 1993, when the AIDS definition was changed, more than 50 percent of the HIV+ women died before they were diagnosed with AIDS. They were not eligible for benefits.

TABLE 4-4   AIDS-Diagnosing OIs (continued)

Symptoms	Comments
sensory loss, tremor, palsy, blindness, personality changes, disorientation, coma. Heart and lung symptoms are also possible.	
Profound involuntary weight loss, inability to absorb nutrients, chronic diarrhea, fever, weakness	This diagnosis is given when other types of infection that could cause weight loss have been ruled out. This is called an exclusionary diagnosis. Chronic weight loss can have a number of primary causes: malnourishment—which can contribute to immune suppression—changes in metabolism, the inability to absorb nutrients, diarrhea, and reduced food intake. The latter, in turn, can result from lack of appetite, oral ulcerations and lesions, and drug side effects.

Myth: If you test negative on the HIV test, you don't have the virus.

Truth: The HIV test looks for the antibodies to HIV, cells produced by the body to defend itself against HIV. Your body usually makes antibodies two weeks to six months, and in some cases even a year, after an infection. In a very small number of cases, the period can be longer. If you want to be as close to certain as you can, have the blood test repeated for at least a year after the possible exposure (i.e., unprotected sex, the sharing of uncleaned needles, needle sticks, etc.). If you want, take the test yearly for a couple of years. Most important, practice safer sex and use your own needle without sharing. These precautions work!

CHAPTER 5

Monitoring Your Treatment

No matter what treatment(s) you and your medical team decide on, monitoring their effectiveness will become your key to survival. Medical personnel are sometimes unaware of all the specific tests available for monitoring immune function. In addition, medical people often interpret results to suit their personal feelings and expectations regarding treatment.

Part of my motivation for writing this book has been to put into your hands all the tools you need for monitoring both your treatments and their effectiveness. There is a long tradition of keeping medical charts and everything on them away from the patients' eyes. This book reverses that tradition, I intend to spell out in detail everything you need to understand your symptoms, lab results, and treatments, and the medical decisions your caregivers make. In the chapters on treatment, I even give you the standards for dosage of prescription drugs as established in the research. Be aware that in doing that I don't mean to suggest that you can go down to your local drugstore and order drugs for self-treatment or am I suggesting that you ignore your doctor's recommendations if they differ from those in this book. I'm simply giving you the detailed information you need to monitor, assess, and interpret your medical situation—the concepts and information that will permit you to ask questions of your medical providers.

Here's an example of a situation in which asking questions

makes all the difference: I have seen clients on AZT who have had initial T4-cell increases, to the enthusiasm of the medical staff. But often, after varying amounts of time, HIV becomes resistant to AZT and T4 cells begin to decline. Certain medical people would say at this point, "It doesn't matter. The rest of your bloodwork looks wonderful."

But the evidence *does* matter. Declining T4 cells and rising P24 antigen levels on AZT are a sign of AZT failure. Where this is the case and the patient's antiviral therapy is not changed, he or she is left with a toxic drug, AZT—a drug that hinders the production of both red and white blood cells—and *no* benefit owing to resistance. Thank goodness, most of the medical world is finally accepting this picture and responding by switching patients to other antiviral therapies. I have been advocating this practice since 1990, and finally, in 1992, studies supporting it were reported at the Eighth International AIDS Conference and mainstream medical providers are beginning this practice.

THE FOUR TREATMENT CATEGORIES

If you understand how to monitor your health, you can intervene early, know if a treatment is effective for *you*, and be prepared for the limitations, if any, of your medical team. But before going into the specifics of monitoring, let's explore the types of treatment interventions available. No matter what modes of treatment you decide on—alternative, holistic, complementary, or mainstream medical—they will fall into one or more of four categories:

1. *antiviral,* a treatment option that will somehow interfere with the HIV virus directly;
2. *immune modulators,* treatments that increase immune response, often increasing T4-cell counts;
3. *OI treatments,* treatments of the specific opportunistic infections (OIs) that are related to HIV infection;
4. *prophylactic treatments,* interventions that *prevent* the occurrence of OIs. When immune markers—signs that indicate the state of the immune system—reach certain levels, people become more susceptible to OIs. Interventions given in response to these markers are called *primary prophylaxis.*

When patients who have had specific OIs are given treatments to prevent recurrence of the conditions, such treatments are called *secondary prophylaxis*.

Treatment plans often include a mixture of these four types of interventions. Anyone on an antiviral should also be using an immune modulator to strengthen and rebuild the immune system. Also, most OIs are preventable, and if you know when to intercede you can often avoid some serious infections. Many of the prophylaxis guidelines are not yet FDA-approved, so health-care providers frequently limit themselves to FDA recommendations. I hope that you will be able to gather as much information as you need to make those decisions yourself or question your health-care professionals until you are comfortable with a given decision.

MONITORING YOUR IMMUNE HEALTH

There are two aspects to effective self-monitoring:

• observing symptoms
• interpreting laboratory studies

Symptom Observation

If your symptoms diminish or go away completely while you are on a specific treatment, that is a sign that, most likely, you do have the targeted opportunistic infection. For example, MAC or MAI, a serious blood infection caused by several mycobacteria, is difficult to diagnose and is often diagnosed too late, after the person is seriously debilitated. But if you have symptoms of MAC (see Table 4-4)* and if your bloodwork indicates that you are in the high-risk category for this OI (T_4 cells under 50 and/or T_4-cell percentage below 5; the difference between absolute number and percentage will be explained later in this chapter), taking the medication, which is relatively nontoxic, and seeing if the symptoms improve would be the basis for a presumptive diagnosis of MAC.

This particular example demonstrates how important it is for you to be observing your own symptoms. With careful symptom observation, you can bring your symptoms to the attention of your medical team *before* you have received a diagnosis. Since patients are often very seriously debilitated by the time MAC is finally detected by blood culture, you will have intervened much earlier, preventing a severely weakened state.

I'd like to take a moment to remind you of a very important fact as you prepare to monitor your symptoms and treatment. People sometimes get colds. People sometimes get the flu. People sometimes get diarrhea. *Not everything is HIV-related!*

Symptom observation is not symptom *obsession*. You can avoid obsession by:

- having a support group
- disclosing, not keeping, secrets
- putting things in perspective through conversation
- keeping a sense of humor, even in the most serious situations

And you can avoid the stress of HIV by:

- having a massage
- taking a run, taking a walk, going to the gym, or doing yoga or some form of exercise—preferably aerobics, which has immune-modulating capabilities (*Note: people who are having trouble gaining weight should avoid these measures*)
- meditating
- counteracting negative thoughts with positive affirmations— for example, instead of saying "I am sick," saying "I am healthy"; instead of saying "I'm dying from," saying "I'm living with"; instead of saying "I am afraid," saying "I am safe." The idea is to believe the most positive thing you can while accepting all possibilities and not obsessing on the negative.

This is a major topic that I'll cover more fully in Chapter 17, The Mind–Body Connection: Psychoneuroimmunology, but I feel it's of prime importance to keep reminding you that your mental attitude is your greatest resource for preserving both your emotional and physical well-being. No matter what's happening, you can gain control over your mind and thoughts and give yourself the greatest gift—peace of mind.

For years, alternative treatment practitioners have drawn attention to the power of the mind over disease—for example, Louise Hay, who claims to have healed her cancer by retraining her mind and emotional responses. Conventional practitioners have gone so far as to recommend that their patients "keep a positive attitude" without ever recommending how or using it as an element in the healing process. Unfortunately, there is sometimes an insincere, patronizing quality to their advice in this area. They are trained in one area to prescribe "strong" medications, which are not always the best solution.

Now, in the area of HIV infection, there exists an extensive scientific study proving the positive effects of exercise and stress reduction. As I mentioned earlier, a University of Miami study of more than 400 HIV+ patients investigated the effects of a regimen of exercise, massage, and stress-reduction meditation/visualization. This was a controlled study, meaning that one group, Group A, did the regimen and a "control" group, B, did not. Group A had a significant rise in T_4 cells and other immune-enhancing cells, but Group B did not. Mary Anne Fletcher, M.D., who conducted the study, stated that the increase in T_4 cells "was about the same as you would expect in the same period if you gave the patients AZT." But when she applied for funds to continue and expand her investigation, the National Institute of Mental Health (NIMH) denied her application. It's unfortunate that the traditional medical community is often unwilling even to explore alternative treatments. However, the National Institutes of Health has recently established a new Office of Alternative Medicine, which will be dedicated to researching the effectiveness of treatments outside of mainstream medicine, including herbal medicine, homeopathy, mind—body techniques and other therapies. Perhaps this office will help to support funding for studies like Dr. Fletcher's.

Now, back to symptom observation. In the case of MAC, it was clear how symptom observation can be a useful tool, but if you are HIV+ and you wait for symptoms before you decide to intervene, you will lose an important advantage—the prevention of HIV progression. Symptom observation is a tool you can use wisely to do the following:

• *judge a treatment's effectiveness, as in the case of MAC;*
• *be able to tell if a treatment* isn't *working.* Case in point: Karen had oral thrush, a yeast infection that causes a white coating, in this case in her mouth. Her doctor prescribed one of the usual treatments for this condition. After a week, her symptoms remained unchanged. Karen did not notify her doctor, thinking the treatment was the only medication available. Depression and feelings of helplessness followed, and the thrush spread down into her esophagus, making it difficult for her to eat. She told no one, enduring in silence, and eventually she was hospitalized for a condition that could have been quickly eradicated by trying an alternative treatment. After extensive testing, it was discovered that Karen had a resistant strain of thrush that responded to other medications. Not only did Karen endure her physical symptoms much longer and more intensely than was necessary, but her emotional anguish intensified because she imagined that her condition was progressing out of control.

• *know if an intervention is needed.* As I mentioned, not every change in health status is HIV-related, though some are. How do you differentiate? Billy, for example, had intense recurrent headaches, which started when he began AZT. When he reported the headaches, the doctor attributed them to AZT and told him they would eventually stop after he adjusted to the drug. But the headaches did not go away, and Billy became used to them. He didn't mention them to the doctor again. While having dinner at his parents' house, Billy had a seizure. He was rushed to the hospital, where he was diagnosed with toxoplasmosis, for which intense recurrent headaches are an early symptom.

Certainly the doctor could have been more active in his follow-up of Billy's condition. But most HIV professionals are overloaded—that is not an excuse, merely a fact—and often miss significant signals. And sometimes patients just aren't persistent enough. If Billy had persisted in mentioning his headaches, the doctor might have ordered a CAT scan or MRI early in the development of this serious OI.

• *help the doctor diagnose an infection.* Charlotte was treated for an ear infection, which the doctor told her was healing well. She also had a sore throat, which she *assumed* was related to the ear and did not mention the additional symptom to her doctor. Charlotte concluded that the throat would stop being sore when the ear healed completely. Finally, she could not swallow, and she came to me, saying, "The doctor is not caring for me correctly. She treated me for an ear infection, which has spread to my throat, and now I can't swallow." After speaking to the doctor, I realized that Charlotte had never mentioned to the doctor that she was having problems with her throat. She turned out to have tonsillitis, which had nothing to do with the ear infection.

Remember to write things down. Try to keep a notepad specifically for doctors' appointments. Writing down symptoms and both time and fever readings can help in the diagnosis of an illness. Report constant headaches, diarrhea, fevers, stomach cramps, coughs, and shortness of breath to your doctor.

Patients often expect doctors to be attentive, alert, and aggressive in asking questions to obtain information. However, doctors often wait for the patient to volunteer information, sometimes on the assumption that mentioning a possibility will create a hypochondriacal complaint.

There is certainly a fine line between symptom observation and symptom obsession. My general rule of thumb is that if it lasts more than one or two days, it is worth reporting. Also, if it is extremely serious the first day, it is worth reporting. The old adage "better safe than sorry" certainly applies here.

Become familiar with your body. You can usually tell when something is seriously wrong—you can "feel" it. Avoid alcohol and drugs, which can mask symptoms.

Finally, becoming familiar with the symptoms of opportunistic infections, by reading books such as this, can help you differentiate between signs of serious infections and the common cold.

The Right Blood Tests and What They Mean

Before we explore each blood test individually, here are some basic guidelines and information regarding when to have blood drawn, how results can differ from lab to lab, and tracking techniques.

• Look for *trends,* not individual numbers. Blood results can vary for many different reasons. Diane's T4-cell count went up and down a hundred points four times over the course of a year (that is, by 100 T4 cells; in discussing T4-cell count, the word *points* is often used to indicate the cells themselves). Basically, she ended the year with the same T4-cell count that she began with. These changes reflected the natural rhythm of her body, and were not a result of HIV infection. All people, HIV+ or HIV−, experience a certain amount of T4-cell count fluctuation over time. If she had known this, Diane could have avoided a lot of emotional distress over the variances in her lab results.

• Have the bloodwork described in this chapter done every three months. Although this is the most effective timetable for following trends, many HIV professionals deviate from it, recommending instead that blood be drawn every six months when T4 cells are well above 500; every three months when T4 cells are between 200 and 500; and more often when T4 cells are below 200. (In this case, a T4-cell count is not always ordered, but other blood results are.)

In contrast, I recommend this timetable for drawing blood and monitoring lab results:

• every three months for T4-cell counts above 300
• more often for T4-cell counts below 300, usually including a T4-cell count

In some cases, results can change drastically and quickly, and keeping a strict eye on lab results makes early intervention possible.

Some people suffer so much emotional stress in anticipating lab results that they have difficulty staying on the every-three-month timetable. If this is the case for you, I recommend that you try to treat your bloodwork as if it were someone else's. Be as objective as possible and respond to bloodwork changes with logical, scientific thinking. Remember, this book is *full* of intervention options for HIV infection.

• Always test at the same time of day. T4-cell counts are lower early in the day and before meals, when fewer T4 cells are circulating than at other times. If your T4 cells are above 600, A.M. to

P.M. variations could be as great as 200 points—which could interfere with the usefulness of comparisons.

• Use the same lab for testing. T4 cells are actually counted by hand. Different labs use different counting techniques and machines, which produce different results. Variations between labs on the East and West coasts can be as great as 200 points in T4-cell counts above 600. (As the count decreases, so does the variation.)

• Avoid testing during periods of infection. Even a minor cold can cause inaccuracies in results. If you are experiencing active symptoms of infection, wait to be tested. Also avoid testing during or after periods of severe stress, recreational drug use (which is not recommended under any circumstances), and lack of sleep.

• Create a chart to track and compare results (see Bloodwork Flowchart, Figure 5-1, page 99).

Let's turn now to the specific tests and test groups.

BLOOD TESTS

The following listing of blood tests is *not* to be used in conjunction with the bloodwork flowchart (Figure 5-1). Below are *test groups* (i.e., the CBC group would include white blood count, red blood count, hemoglobin, hematocrit, and others). These test-group names are used by the doctor to order labwork. When you speak with your doctor regarding the ordering of bloodwork, or if you can make your own order, you would use these test-group names, as listed on the lab form. This section is an overview of test groups, individual tests, and their use. Later in the chapter, I will cover in more detail individual tests in the order that they appear on the bloodwork flowchart (Figure 5-1).

• CBC (complete blood count)—a breakdown of the red and white blood cell counts
• complete lymphocyte test (lymphocyte phenotyping)—an overview of the immune cells. This includes the T4-cell (other terms are CD4, helper, and T cell) count and percentage, the T8-cell (other terms are CD8 or suppressor cell) count and percent-

age, and the CD_4/CD_8 ratio (a comparison of the balance of T_4 and T_8 cells)

• ESR or sedimentation rate—a count that rises with active infection; not HIV-specific, but high levels (above 40) have been associated with HIV infection

• platelet count—measures the clotting factor, which stops bleeding, and is sometimes depleted by HIV

• SMAC chemistry panel—general tests providing an overview of organ function

• amylase level—increased amylase can signal pancreas problems; important for people on the antiviral ddI

• beta-2 microglobulin—a protein that usually rises prior to the appearance of HIV-related symptoms in HIV+ people

• neopterin level—a protein level elevated by HIV progression; some doctors believe this test is interchangeable with beta-2 microglobulin

• albumin—the level of protein in the blood; below-normal levels are an indicator of HIV progression

• P24 antigen and P24 antibody (for political reasons, these tests are not commercially available in every state, but blood can be sent out to labs in California or New Jersey to be tested for these levels; see Resource Guide)—protein 24 (P24) is the core of the HIV virus. P24 antigen supposedly measures levels of virus, but has not shown significant correlation with disease progression. P24 antibody measures the level of antibodies, infection-fighting cells, specific to HIV, which are an indication of the immune system's efficiency in controlling the HIV virus. Some doctors believe that when the P24 antibody count is above 1,000, the chances of developing symptoms are lowered.

OTHER TESTS

These tests are not necessarily done by blood sample. They are other testing procedures that can help you measure your immune status and your exposure to other HIV-related infections. These tests are useful in deciding on preventive or prophylaxis therapies (see Chapter 14, Preventive Therapy).

• anergy panel—a measure of immune response. Small amounts of infectious proteins are injected under the skin. If the immune system is strong, the area will welt or blow up from an immune response. A special tool is used to measure the size of the welts; the larger the welt, the stronger the immune response. However, if the immune system is weakened, there may be no welting response.

• TB test (PPD)—tests for tuberculosis, which is epidemic among HIV+ people and should be tested for at least once a year. In this test, a small amount of TB is injected under the skin to determine whether or not the person has been exposed to mycobacterium tuberculosis (TB). If the immune system is weakened, there may be no way to determine by this test if you have been exposed to TB. Therefore, the anergy panel is necessary along with the PPD to make certain that the immune system is still mounting a response (this practice was recommended in a study at the Eighth International AIDS Conference in Amsterdam, 1992: PoB 3088). No response on the anergy panel would suggest that the immune system was weakened, but a negative PPD would not conclusively rule out TB exposure. In such a case, sputum samples and chest X rays would be ordered.

• baseline toxoplasmosis titer—if positive, measures the amount of *Toxoplasma gondii,* the infectious agent for this opportunistic brain infection. If the baseline test is positive, taking regular titers will indicate the need for treatment or prevention before the infection has progressed to a symptomatic stage. For this infection, titers are followed more closely if T4 cells go below 100 or to 5 percent (percent is calculated by measuring the number of T4 cells in relation to other kinds of immune system cells, lymphocytes, in the body)—that is when symptoms of toxoplasmosis infection are at the highest risk of manifesting.

• hepatitis B—if negative, consider the hepatitis B vaccination.

• baseline CMV titer—most HIV+ people have been exposed to cytomegalovirus (CMV). This infection is found often undiagnosed upon autopsy. The current theory suggests that underlying CMV is much more common than the diagnosed cases, and untreated it speeds up HIV progression. To avoid this, CMV prophylaxis treatment is recommended, especially if regular titers show a rise and T4 cells are dropping. Use natural prophylaxis for 200–500 T4-cell counts (see Chapter 8); for T4-cell counts under 200, aggressive medical prophylaxis is recommended (Chapter 14).

• parasite, yeast, and fungus stool sample—potentially

chronic, underlying infections that usually put undue stress on the immune system. Most people have been exposed to these infections. I recommend herbal treatments that target them for anyone who is HIV+ (see Chapter 8). Everyone should have these tests once, no matter what the T-cell level.

• MAI screen/MAC screen (the terms are used interchangeably)—to test for this opportunistic infection. When T4 cells are below 100, blood-culture and sputum tests for MAC are recommended every three months. If negative, consider prophylaxis (Chapter 14).

TESTS SPECIFIC TO WOMEN

The needs of the HIV+ woman differ from those of men, which is why Chapter 11 is devoted solely to women's concerns. Gynecological problems are extremely common in HIV+ women, and regular OB-GYN visits for the following procedures are recommended:

• Pap smear—a monitoring tool for conditions affecting the cervix (the tip of the uterus). Recommended every three to six months. HIV+ women sometimes have irregular Pap smears with no apparent cause. Colposcopy, a more reliable test of the cervix, is recommended.

• Colposcopy—a device that magnifies the tissue of the cervix under a bright light up to 40 times. Usually combined with a biopsy, the examination tests a small tissue sample for cell changes or cancerous cells.

• Routine vaginal exam—for detecting yeast or other infections, which are easily treated.

SAMPLE BLOODWORK

Figure 5-1 (see page 99) is a sample (blank) bloodwork flowchart that shows how to track specific results of the blood tests. Figure 5-2 (see pages 100–101) consists of two actual labwork samples, and a bloodwork flowchart. On the labwork, I've circled the names of the tests, the results, and the normal ranges for these results so that you can see how to transfer results from labwork to your flowchart. I have filled in the sample flowchart with the lab results and have indicated corresponding test results transferred to the flowchart with a series of circled numbers (1–14). Make sure you discuss with your medical provider any results outside the normal range. Ask questions about anything you see on your lab results that is not explained in this book. Remember, "Don't worry about it" or "Oh, that's nothing" is not an answer; it is an avoidance. When you get those reactions, ask for clarification.

YOUR BLOOD FLOWCHART

Using Figure 5-1 as a model (consider photocopying it), keep a record of your own bloodwork results. In Figure 5-2, I have filled in the results from the sample. Follow this along as I explain what to look for in each separate result. Note that in this sample labwork and flowchart, you will not see reference ranges for the following tests as they were not ordered for this particular patient: WBC (white blood count); ESR (sedimentation rate); P24 antigen, P24 antibody, and neopterin. The WBC, in particular, is a major result needed for measuring HIV progression. It is important to be aware of your doctor's instructions to the lab so that you can make sure you are receiving the necessary tests. (The circled numbers next to the test names correspond to the numbers in the flowchart.)

• **WBC** (white blood count)—All the cells of the immune system are white blood cells. You must refer to the reference range on your own labwork, since your results will correlate with the range set by your lab. Neutropenia, the depletion of a common type of white blood cell, is sometimes seen in patients on AZT. Immune modulators can increase white-blood-cell counts.

• **RBC** (1) (red blood count), **HGB** (2) (hemoglobin), **HCT** (3) (hematocrit)—These tests are interrelated and measure the cells that function primarily to transport oxygen within the body. When HGB and HCT fall below the normal level, this is an early sign of anemia, which ultimately could also deplete RBC.

Triglycerides (4)—Measurements of triglycerides, fatty acids in the body, have been found to be abnormally high in up to a third of AIDS patients and many HIV+ patients as well. High triglyceride levels can indicate excessive activity of TNF, tumor

FIGURE 5-1.   Bloodwork Flowchart

Test Name	Date	Date	Date	Date	Date	Date	Date	Date
WBC								
RBC								
HGB								
HCT								
Triglycerides								
Albumin								
Platelets								
ESR or sed rate								
T4 %								
T4 #								
T8 %								
T8 #								
CD4/CD8 ratio								
Beta-2 micro-globulin								
P24 antigen								
P24 antibody								
Neopterin								
SGOT								
SGPT								

FIGURE 5-2 Labwork Samples

LAB A

(1) TEST	(2) RESULTS ABNORMAL	(2) NORMAL	(3) REFERENCE RANGE	(4) UNITS
⑤ ALBUMIN		4.7	3.9–5.5	GM/DL
GLUCOSE	57 L		65–120	MG/DL
UREA NITROGEN		18	6–27	MG/DL
CREATININE		1.0	0.5–1.6	MG/DL
CHOLESTEROL		189	130–200	MG/DL
④ TRIGLYCERIDES		91	30–180	MG/DL
URIC ACID		4.8	3.2–8.4	MG/DL
TOTAL BILI.		0.6	0.0–1.2	MG/DL
ALK. PHOS.		85	40–150	MU/ML
LDH		201	60–290	MU/ML
⑬ SGOT (AST)		29	1–50	MU/ML
⑭ SGPT (ALT)		32	1–50	MU/ML

LAB B

(1) TEST NAME	(2) RESULTS	(4) UNITS	(3) REFERENCE RANGE
① RBC	4.89	MIL./CU.MM	4.50–5.90
② HGB	16.30	GM/DL	13.5–17.6
③ HCT	47.60	PERCENT	40.0–52.0
MCV	97.00	FL	83.0–103
MCHC	34.20	PERCENT	31.0–37.0
RDW	15.90	PERCENT	12.0–16.2
MPV	8.90	FL	6.90–11.4
⑥ PLATELET COUNT	171.00	THOUS./CU.MM	140–440
⑫ BETA2MICROGLOBULIN'S	2.10	MG/L	.70–3.40

****

TEST OR TEST GROUP WITH A VALUE OUTSIDE THE ESTABLISHED REFERENCE RANGE

IMMUNE COMPETENCE	* (01)		
TOTAL B-LYMPH			
CD20 (6.0 PCT)	61.00	CU.MM	55– 622
TOTAL T-LYMPH			
CD2 (91.0 PCT)	937.00	CU.MM	967–2419
T-LYMPH SUBSETS			
CD4 ⑦(12.0 PCT)	⑧ 123.00	CU.MM	537–1571
CD8 ⑨(70.0 PCT)	⑩ 721.00	CU.MM	235– 753
⑪ CD4/CD8	0.17	RATIO	1.20–3.80

"Ratio" is another name for this test

T4-cell "absolute" number

T4-cell percent

Asterisk line—Lab B lists all tests outside the reference range below this line. This can be troublesome. Tests are listed in order—Lab B disregards the order for "abnormal" results, making them difficult to find.

This is your T4-cell count

Sample Flowchart

	DATE BLOOD WAS TAKEN
WBC N/A	N/A — REFERENCE RANGE / RESULT
① RBC 4.50-5.90	4.89
② HGB 13.5-17.6	16.3
③ HCT 40.0-52.0	47.6
④ Triglycerides 30-180	91
⑤ Albumin 3.9-5.5	4.7
⑥ Platelets 140-440	171.0
ESR or sed rate N/A	N/A
⑦ T₄ N/A %	12.0%
⑧ T₄ 537-1571 #	123
⑨ T₈ N/A %	70%
⑩ T₈ 235-753 #	721
⑪ CD₄/CD₈ ratio 1.20-3.80	0.17
⑫ Beta-2 micro-globulin	2.10
P₂₄ antigen N/A	N/A
P₂₄ antibody N/A	N/A
Neopterin N/A	N/A
⑬ SGOT 1-50	29
⑭ SGPT 1-50	32

N/A—Not available

Figure 5-2. Labwork sample. This figure consists of two samples of labwork results (labeled Lab A and Lab B), similar to the reports you can get from your doctor. As you can see, the formats differ from each other—and both might differ from yours—but the information is listed in a similar way. Most labwork will have these four categories: (1) "Test" (the name of the test); (2) "Results," the numbers you are concerned about (some labs, such as A, have "abnormal" and "normal" columns; others, like B, list abnormal results below the asterisk line); (3) "Reference Range" is the "normal range." Ideally you would like your results to fall within this range; those that don't will be in the "abnormal" column; (4) "Units" is the mathematical value of the result.

necrosis factor (an immune system protein), which can increase HIV replication, cause wasting syndrome, and almost completely reverse the antiretroviral effect of the drugs AZT, ddC, and ddI. Since TNF can interfere with absorption, it is possible that nutrient intake and effectiveness of any stomach-digested treatment would be reduced. One treatment option that reduced triglyceride levels dramatically was Trental (see Chapter 10, Antiviral Options).

• **Albumin** (5)—A protein measurement of the blood. According to a study presented at the Amsterdam conference (PoB 3695), each .5-gm/dL decrease in albumin was a significant decline, definitely related to HIV progression (this is discussed further in Chapter 15, Nutrition and HIV). In addition, this level is used to measure wasting syndrome, an AIDS-defining syndrome where a person loses 10 percent of his or her body weight for no apparent reason. Protein is the element the body uses to make new cells. A good albumin level could improve the chances of other counts returning to or staying within the normal range.

• **Platelet count** (6)—This test measures the number of cells available to help stop bleeding. Idiopathic thrombocytopenia purpura (ITP; low platelets) is a condition that is common in HIV+ people and is easily reversed early on.

• **ESR** (sedimentation or sed rate)—this test measures how quickly red blood cells settle. The rate will rise with active infection, though not necessarily HIV-infection specific. However, high sed rates have been associated with HIV infection.

• **T4-** (or CD4-) **cell count** (7) and **percentage** (8)—There are two important aspects of T4-cell counts, the absolute count and the percentage. Although the reference range for this count differs from lab to lab, there are range categories specific to HIV infection. When an HIV+ person has an absolute count of 500 or above, the likelihood of developing symptoms is extremely low. Most OIs develop when T cells are below 200, but as in all aspects of HIV infection, the measurements are far from 100-percent predictive. Many people with fewer than 200 T cells remain asymptomatic. A good friend of mine, Tom, has had an absolute count of 20 T cells for five years now, and is still asymptomatic. Look around, talk to people, and you'll run across many similar stories. There are no real statistics on what percentage of people develop OIs when they reach 200 T4 cells, but from personal experience, I believe it is lower than 50 percent. The percentage is a measurement of T4 cells in relation to other immune system cells in the body. The body has a balance which it struggles to maintain. The T4-cell percentage reflects a measurement of that balance.

The T4-cell percentage was once used by public health officials as an indicator for prophylaxis. At 20 percent, PCP prophylaxis was recommended; at 5 percent, other prophylaxis was deemed appropriate. But the U.S. Public Health Service Task Force has now changed the guidelines for PCP prophylaxis; now this practice is recommended when the absolute T4-cell count (the count without the percentage indicator) is below 200–250. See Chapter 14 for specific recommendations.

• **T8** (9, 10)—These cells, the suppressor cells that shut down the immune system, are also given in total count and percentage of total T cells. Early on in the HIV pandemic, researchers theorized that an abundance of T8 cells would constantly shut down an already compromised immune system. Since then, however, many HIV physicians have noted that people with high T8-cell counts remain asymptomatic even when T4 cells decline. Some have speculated that T8 cells adjust and begin doing the work of T4 cells. But an article in *BETA* (August 1992) noted that CD8 cells (also known as T8 cells) attack HIV-infected cells, killing them or suppressing viral replication. The report indicated that CD8 cells released cytokines, which are intercellular messengers. A previously undiscovered cytokine stops HIV replication in test-tube-grown cells. With this evidence, the theory of T8 cells' somehow helping to maintain wellness seems verified.

• **CD4/CD8 ratio** (T4/T8 ratio) (11)—If the ratio is going down, you will have an abundance of suppressor cells. As explained above, this is not necessarily a negative development, but one study noted an increase in symptom development when ratios drop below .25. The size of the increase was not specified.

• **Beta-2 microglobulin** (12)—This is probably one of the most important tests for measuring HIV progression. It is easy to perform and one study found it superior to P24-antigen or T4 count in predicting disease progression. When T4 cells are ruptured, which probably means that HIV has replicated within the cell, beta-2, a surface protein, is released into the bloodstream. One study showed that with beta-2 results over 5.0, the risk of serious opportunistic infection more than doubled. Most HIV professionals agree that results under 3.0 are good, between 3.0 and 5.0 are midrange, and above 5.0 are high. These are, again, HIV-specific indicators. If your intervention is working, this number should be going down. Antiviral interventions would affect this number. Two small European studies show that a history of IV drug use may affect this level and therefore diminish its usefulness. I still recommend using the number as part of the complete picture and relying more heavily on the neopterin level, which many practitioners feel is interchangeable with the beta-2 microglobulin.

• **P24 antigen**—The results of this test are currently inconclusive, but it is continually used in HIV research, with a decreasing number indicating treatment efficacy. A correlation between this measurement and HIV progression is questionable. The P24 antigen is typically measured in volume by rising numbers. Often the results of this test are given in negative and positive terms— "you're P24 negative" or "you're P24 positive," period. But it's more important to know the direction of the absolute P24 count than whether you're negative or positive in any one lab report. For example, you can be P24 "positive" at 100 and 80, but the antigen number is decreasing, which is a positive sign. Track the direction of results of this test over time. If your treatment is effective, the result should be falling.

• **P24 antibody**—The theory is that these are the antibodies to HIV, so the higher the antibody count, the more effectively your immune system is responding to HIV, so the chance of becoming sick decreases. P24 antigen and antibody are tests created specifically for HIV infection, measuring the P24 in HIV. Results above 1,000 are very good, above 200 are okay, and below 200 are considered low. If you are taking immune modulators, this test result should be increasing, and this would be the trend to try to maintain.

• **Neopterin**—As with beta-2 microglobulin, elevated neopterin levels are linked to HIV disease progression. Many physicians believe that it's redundant to monitor both beta-2 and neopterin, since studies show them to be equally accurate predictors. But for people who, because of collapsed veins, have difficulty in giving blood samples, measuring neopterin levels is a useful option, since they can be measured in urine. In addition, none of these tests are definitively conclusive, so all the information that shows some efficacy should be used to get as close as possible to a sound clinical prediction. If you're tracking the effectiveness of an antiviral intervention, you'll be looking for the neopterin level to decrease. New studies emanating from the Eighth International AIDS Conference cite neopterin as "the single marker rising consistently with the progression of HIV disease." In summary, an increasing neopterin level would indicate HIV progression.

• **SGOT** (13) and **SGPT** (14)—These tests measure liver enzymes, and since many HIV drugs (including AZT and Tagamet) cause liver toxicity, it's important to follow these levels to avoid liver damage. Also, ex-alcoholics and substance abusers might have elevated liver-enzyme levels; they can take natural interventions to try to help normalize these values (see Chapter 8).

No single test mentioned here is a great predictor *on its own* of HIV disease progression or treatment effectiveness. But an overview of *all* these levels can give you a good idea of your immune status and whether a treatment regimen is working or needs modification. The tests I've described measure the immune system and HIV progression specifically. If most of the levels are moving in the correct direction, your treatment regimen is probably working. Remember, you're taking an overview and looking for general trends, so even if one or two results have dropped slightly or remained the same, if the others have shown significant increases, the news is good. And being stable—with your numbers the same from quarter to quarter—is a good sign.

In addition to results of the tests I have outlined, discuss with your medical caregiver *any* result on your bloodwork that is not in the reference range. Ask what the test is related to, if the result is serious, and how to rectify the result if necessary.

Whenever you have blood drawn, you pay for that bloodwork, and most doctors supply copies of the reports upon request without incident. Legally, in most states, the doctor must supply you with a written summary upon request. If you are making a commitment to yourself to participate in your HIV treatment as fully as possible, you are also making a commitment to monitor your bloodwork. Without monitoring your bloodwork and symptoms, it's difficult to tell if a treatment regimen is working.

One short story to wrap up this chapter shows the value of this sort of detailed self-observation and participation: Cecelia had been on AZT for two years. Her T_4 cells had consistently dropped over the last three quarterly blood tests. She was not getting a beta-2, but her white blood count was declining and her T_4/T_8 ratio was falling. Her doctor was a great believer in AZT therapy, and interpreted these results as fine as long as Cecelia was not developing symptoms. I disagreed and recommended she change her antiviral therapy from AZT to ddI. She was afraid of her doctor and did not change. One year later, she was extremely ill and in the hospital. Her doctor came to her and advised her to change to ddI.

HIV is a disease of *prevention*. Cecelia's progression was quite probably preventable. The blood results clearly indicated a need for a change in antiviral therapy, and that change early on could have prevented the progression of Cecelia's illness and kept her out of the hospital.

Your bloodwork is your key to understanding your treatment choices. It will reflect effectiveness—and tell you when it's time to change. Focusing on the numbers and their direction gives you real, indisputable, black-and-white evidence on which to base your treatment decisions. Combined with symptom observation and a continuing education into available options, it forms the basis for your full participation in your medical decision-making.

BREAKING THE MYTHS

Myth: Only the doctor has the right to read and interpret bloodwork results.
Truth: You paid for them. Asking for a copy is a reasonable request. In most states, you are legally entitled to copies, upon request.

Myth: It's psychologically destructive for you to know the ups and downs of your test levels.
Truth: The truth empowers you, makes it possible for you to make decisions, and alleviates the sense of helplessness and hopelessness that you get when you turn over your life decisions to somebody else.

Myth: HIV infection manifests itself the same way in both sexes.

Truth: Many gynecological problems are related to HIV in women.

Myth: T4 cells are the be-all and end-all measurement of HIV progression.

Truth: T4 cells are one measurement in a total picture composed of the results discussed in this chapter.

PART II

TREATMENT OPTIONS

CHAPTER 6

The Range of Treatment Options

This is the chapter and the section of the book that most of my readers have been waiting for: here's where I survey the treatment options that are available to treat HIV infection. I am certain that many readers have picked up this book just to read this section, but if you've flipped directly to this page, please be aware that this section is built on the information preceding it. I can't emphasize enough the importance of the material covered in Chapters 1 through 5.

Look once more at the preceding chapter where I discuss learning to monitor your labwork for the effectiveness of your treatment option or options, and you'll understand what I mean. If you are still unclear about any of the material in Chapter 5 on monitoring your bloodwork, I urge you to reread the chapter, because I will consistently refer back to the information on bloodwork. If you don't have that foundation, what you learn about treatments in this and subsequent chapters will be less useful and valuable to you.

TYPES OF TREATMENT OPTIONS

The available treatment options for HIV infection break down
into three categories:

- mainstream medical treatment options (also called traditional therapies)
- complementary therapies
- alternative therapies

Mainstream, or traditional, therapies are those therapies your
doctor is most likely to prescribe. These are treatments that have
been approved specifically for HIV infection by the Food and
Drug Administration, the FDA. Some current examples include
AZT, ddI, ddC, and even alpha interferon, pentamidine, and
Bactrim. All these therapies have been approved by the FDA for
the treatment of HIV infection.

The distinction between complementary and alternative treatments often becomes blurred, but I define *complementary* therapies as those that would probably be less threatening to many
doctors than alternative therapies and that can coexist with traditional treatments. My experience with doctors tells me that the
term *complementary* is easier for them to accept—and *any* additional treatment can be complementary.

Complementary therapies may be drugs that the FDA has
not *yet* approved for HIV infection but that are approved for another use and that show significant efficacy in the treatment of
specific aspects of HIV infection. In such a case, the prescriptions
doctors write for the treatment are called *off-label* prescriptions.
Off-label prescription writing is very common in everyday medical practice—almost 60 percent of the prescriptions written in
the United States are for off-label uses.

Complementary treatments, then, include such therapies as,
for example, the appetite stimulants Megace and Marinol, which
have not been approved as appetite stimulants in HIV infection,
but have been studied, have shown some efficacy, and are being
widely used in that capacity. Complementary treatments might
also include some vitamins, probably the more common ones,
such as B_{12} shots, and those that are available by prescription
rather than the vitamins used routinely in alternative regimens.

The last category, *alternative treatments,* is often frowned upon by the medical community. These are treatments such as diet regimens, herbs, and vitamin supplements. This category encompasses many, many practices, including acupuncture, chiropractic, Chinese herbology, and massage.

In my work with people infected with HIV, I try not to judge anyone's treatment choice. Rather, I focus on my clients' baseline bloodwork—where people start—and then see if they improve or not under the treatments they are taking. This is the precise approach I'm advocating here: Learn what's out there, participate fully in choosing your treatments, and then monitor your bloodwork for bottom-line evidence of the effectiveness—or efficacy—of those treatments.

That approach is fundamental to this book, my practice, and my underlying orientation. If you decide on a treatment regimen, whatever it may be, and if your bloodwork is not improving—and certainly the way you feel is a major part of measuring treatment efficacy, but your subjective feelings must be backed up by concrete bloodwork results—I would recommend that you keep changing your treatment options until you find something that does have a positive effect on your lab results.

Alternative treatments have also been called *holistic* (also spelled *wholistic*). To me, this word means addressing the mind, the body, and the spirit—the *whole* person—with your treatment regimen. Now, this seems like a good idea whether you're doing traditional, complementary, *or* alternative treatments. So in this book I use the word *holistic* to encompass *all* these treatment regimens, plus additional techniques such as meditation, stress reduction, acupuncture, herbology, acupressure, homeopathy, deep breathing, and massage.

Many practitioners and medical writers in the United States describe Western medicine in just this way—as addressing the mind, body, and spirit, and treating the *whole person* rather than just the disease (if you accept the term *disease*). And yet once inside the examining room, very few physicians ask, "How are you doing today? Any major changes in your life this month or around the time that you got sick?" Although the holistic way has been heralded as *the* way to practice medicine, it is not the way routine medicine is practiced. Most physicians today are usually too busy, or their communicating and socializing skills are inadequate, to really address the whole person. And doctors are often overwhelmed by their own feelings regarding HIV infection, which are frequently intertwined with loss, grief, and fear. Since most work independently, despite a hospital setting or office practice, they have little or no opportunity to process these feelings, a requirement for good emotional health that is often impossible to meet alone. Their unresolved feelings make it impossible for them to deliver the kind of comprehensive care we all hope for. And often their own unexpressed and unprocessed grief comes through to patients in the form of negative and even fatalistic messages. The point is not to blame doctors for not being trained in these areas, but to empower yourself to deal with their deficiencies.

Yet the need to deal with illness holistically is so fundamental that, in my opinion, it is simply the *only* way to proceed. It's for just this reason that you yourself need to be at the helm of your medical team. Although it's possible that you will luck out with your medical caregivers and find one or some whose approach is truly holistic, it is ultimately up to you to make sure that your treatment regimen embraces not just your physical being but your mental and spiritual ones as well.

Such a multifaceted program means that you will be drawing from all three categories of options—mainstream, complementary, and alternative—as you need them to round out a true holistic regimen. Drawing freely from the whole universe of medical and psychological/spiritual options and integrating them in this way will give you a custom-designed, person-centered treatment regimen.

AN INTEGRATED APPROACH

Integrating options means expanding your knowledge of the many possible therapies so you can personalize your treatment program and mold it to your specific character as well as your physical needs.

Your mental and spiritual conditions are as much a part of HIV infection as the virus that has entered your body. In the Western Hemisphere, with a few exceptions, this part of medicine has been ignored.

Not so many years ago—in the thirties, forties, and even fifties—doctors asked personal questions as part of the examination routine. If you read your physician's notes, you would have seen there, "Lost his job," "Broke up with his wife," or "Seems dejected but unwilling to discuss." These weren't idle observations from a slower, more easygoing era; they entered the medical record because they were considered significant to the treatment process.

But as medicine became more informed, it also became more narrow-minded. It took something like HIV to come along and shake people, waking them up to the fact that there might be different ways of approaching healing than just prescribing a pill. This is an aspect of medicine that has been rediscovered, and much of that rediscovery is due to HIV infection.

THE MODES OF INTERVENTION

As you design your very specific treatment regimen to match your physical needs, values and beliefs, temperament, and spiritual concerns, you will also want to be aware that the traditional, complementary, and alternative treatments will fit into one of the four intervention modes that I mentioned in Chapter 5:

- antivirals, a treatment option that will somehow interfere with the HIV virus directly
- immune modulators, treatments that increase the body's immune response, often resulting in a T_4-cell increase
- OI treatments, treatments for specific opportunistic infection related to HIV
- prophylactic treatments, treatments that prevent the occurrence of OIs

As a person trying to develop a treatment plan, it is important that you understand and choose from these modes of intervention. This is not something to leave up to your doctor; it's an important aspect that you should understand, help create, and participate in monitoring. You might want to integrate one or even several options from *each* of these categories—or at least from two of these categories, depending on your current bloodwork and symptoms. I am careful about making general statements, and usually hate to do so, but for people with T_4 cells above 500–600—or some people would rather do this at an even higher count, above 700 or 800—a good place to begin is with the less toxic, more natural treatment interventions (to be discussed fully in Chapter 8). Careful monitoring will tell you if they are working in either sustaining you and suppressing HIV progression, or rebuilding you to an even higher T4-cell count.

CALIBRATING THE AGGRESSIVENESS OF YOUR TREATMENT

If your T4 cells were above, say, 700 and consistently dropping, you might want to try some of the more aggressive but relatively nontoxic treatments, such as immune modulators. The most commonly used medical immune modulators are Tagamet, Antabuse, and naltrexone, and these three drugs work best when your T4 cells are above 250. These drugs, which fall into the midrange on a measure of aggressiveness, often build up the T4-cell count. When I use the term *aggressive* to describe interventions, in my mind it denotes treatments that work more quickly but with a greater risk of side effects and toxicity than the less aggressive approaches. So in effect the most aggressive treatment would also be the most toxic.

The very aggressive drugs—those *I* consider very aggressive—are my last choice. These are AZT, ddI, and ddC. I recommend using these drugs as a last resort and in a very limited capacity.

EVALUATING YOUR OPTIONS: GENERAL GUIDELINES

In the above paragraphs, I've given you my own personal opinions regarding treatment aggressiveness and the balancing of options. When I discuss individual drugs, I'll cover many of the opinions, theories, and philosophies surrounding them, not just my own. It will be up to you to decide what's best for you. These decisions are often difficult, and I know some people would prefer to have an "expert" take them by the hand and take control of their treatment regimens. But, as I have established by now, handing over control is dangerous, and in HIV infection there are few, if any, complete experts. Try to work with a team of support group members, alternative treatment professionals, an

HIV therapist, a good mainstream practitioner, and several others of your own choice.

- If you remain in control and make the decisions, you have the power.
- When you let someone else make the treatment decisions, you are truly powerless, and that feeling of powerlessness can induce or reinforce depression and a sense of being out of control.
- Your team of professionals can help you make a decision.

But rest assured that in taking control and making your own decisions, you won't be entering the unknown without a guide:

- *Follow your bloodwork* and the answers will be there for you.

Should you continue on a regimen when your T4 cells have dropped 200 points? There would have to be a very good reason to continue.

Should you continue on a regimen when your T4 count has remained at the same point? Maybe. Evidence of no HIV progression is definitely a plus. But if the T cells have remained the same and the beta-2 microglobulin, which is released into the bloodstream when T4 cells are ruptured, has gone up significantly, it is possible that the immune-modulation portion of your regimen is working and the antiviral part is not.

Remember, the T4-cell count often reflects the effect of *both* antivirals and immune modulators, whereas the beta-2 blood test would reflect the effect of your antiviral alone. So, if you are combining different options, you'll need to make these kinds of distinctions, learning which drugs have an effect on which measurements, in order to evaluate their efficacy.

Note, too, that the more natural treatment interventions usually take longer to work than mainstream approaches. If a natural-treatment intervention doesn't work after three months, I would definitely give it more time. Most natural-treatment interventions take six months to a year to show results. If you don't have the time wait for those results, you should be on a more aggressive treatment, boosting your cells, controlling HIV, and *then* substituting the more natural treatments.

Usually, when T4 cells have fallen below 200, I suggest aggressive treatment (e.g., AZT) to build the immune system *first*. Then, with more natural treatment options supporting the new buildup, I recommend eliminating the aggressive toxic therapies. This approach is supported by a recent study reported at the Eighth International AIDS Conference in 1992 (PoB 3669), in which participants on AZT—four weeks on, four weeks off— had fewer opportunistic infections and greater stabilization of T4-cell increases than those on daily AZT therapy.

My suggestion goes one step further: hold off on toxic therapies until blood values indicate they are needed. When your T4 cells are above 350, there is a low risk of developing an opportunistic infection, so waiting for an alternative treatment or more natural treatment to work might be the way to avoid the need for a more aggressive, more toxic treatment intervention. If T4 cells continue to decline to below 300, it is still early enough to use a drug such as AZT and gain benefit, usually evidenced by a rise in T4-cell count.

There are varying opinions within the medical establishment as to whether early intervention with AZT, when T4 cells are at 500, is the best treatment advice.

THINGS YOU NEED TO KNOW

When I discuss individual treatment options in this book, I usually use the brand name, which is a registered trademark name the drug company comes up with, followed by the generic scientific name in parentheses (see section title on page 142, for example). I usually use the most common "street" name throughout the discussion. Your care provider will understand either name when you mention it in discussions of your treatment. (See page 142 for more details.)

Another term will come up often in the following chapters to describe a "new" way to prescribe medications: *prophylaxis*. This term is used very commonly in the field of HIV infection to indicate that a treatment is being used not as a *response* to a particular infection, but as a preventive before it occurs.

CRITERIA FOR CHOOSING OPTIONS

Recently, I've gotten back bloodwork on seven clients, and all of their reports showed significant positive changes. Each of these people has a different treatment regimen. My approach to designing regimens breaks down into three stages:

- If a person has a T4-cell count below 200, I begin with very aggressive treatments, such as AZT, ddI, ddC, or d4T, rebuilding and slowly adding the more natural regimens.
- There's a midpoint, between 200 and 350, where I take away the very toxic regimens but am still putting in aggressive treatments—like Tagamet, naltrexone, and Peptide T, an antiviral I will talk about at length—and adding more natural interventions. This phase will continue until T4 cells are approximately 500.
- In the third phase, when T4 cells are above 500, I'll take away the more aggressive therapies and leave people with the most natural therapies, which will take them the rest of the way and maintain them.

I advised one client to switch from AZT to ddI, and his T cells went up 300 points, from 150 to 450. At that point I stopped the ddI, replacing it with other treatments that were somewhat less aggressive. I don't believe that at that range you need to use the most toxic, aggressive medications. Again, this decision reflected my personal opinion, which suited the patient's own needs and temperament.

Now, many doctors and the FDA would say that if you're on ddI or AZT and it's working, stay on it forever. I disagree, because research shows that those drugs stop working after a time, and when that happens—I'll discuss this in detail when I focus on the specific drugs in later chapters—you're just taking in toxicity without benefit; this could be very harmful.

For example, Frank began AZT treatment with 600 T cells and eight months later had 90. Such a significant drop in T cells would be unusual even if he had been on no medication at all. But the HIV virus becomes resistant to AZT, which has been well documented, and when that happens T cells can drop quickly. The extreme rapidity of Frank's T-cell decrease was highly unusual, but in many cases, the dramatic T-cell drop-off occurs in people who are kept on toxic, aggressive drugs long after they have become resistant.

I'm telling stories like Frank's to illustrate that it is important to remain flexible—to know that even the most natural treatment now working for you might stop working someday. At that point, it would be counterproductive to hold on to the known treatment, telling yourself, "No, it worked in the past; it will work again." Even the best regimens often stop working after a period, which can be very successful in boosting immune stamina. Remain flexible. There are enough options out there to allow you to change your routine and remain healthy. Don't shortchange yourself by becoming stuck in one particular treatment regimen.

At the risk of repeating myself, I should stress the fact that the need to stay flexible and open to change only reinforces the importance of knowing how to

- read your bloodwork
- and monitor it regularly.

Frank had some blood tests, and he saw his T_4 cells dropping, but unfortunately his doctor insisted on continuing AZT therapy, even when these results suggested AZT failure. And he knew no better.

Another client, Diane, was also on AZT, and her doctor excitedly told her, "Your T_4 cells have gone up. Isn't that great?" With the next lab report, her T_4 cells had gone up again, and her doctor said, "Your T_4 cells have gone up *again*! Isn't that wonderful?" But in another three months, Diane's T_4 cells had gone down, and the doctor said, "Oh, it doesn't mean anything. The rest of your bloodwork looks great." Now, why did it mean something when the count was going up and mean nothing when it was going down?

Since HIV treatment options are often very limited, doctors can get caught in their own frustration and refuse to consider other options. When T_4 cells go down, this might be a sign that an intervention is not working. Remember, if the T-cell level declines slightly and then goes right back up, there really is nothing to worry about. But if the declines are significant—more than 50 T_4 cells, or several T_4-cell declines over a period of months—then it is time to look at a new treatment regimen.

* * *

To summarize, complementary, alternative, and traditional treatment options will all fit into the four treatment modes: antiviral, immune modulator, opportunistic infection treatments, or prophylaxis. You will often combine an immune modulator and an antiviral, depending on the way they work in your body. Understanding how a drug works in the body is an important factor in putting together a treatment regimen. You don't want different options that overlap and have the same mechanisms of action. You want to be choosing treatments with different mechanisms of action so you're not taking in extra medications doing the same job. For instance, you might combine the antiviral AZT with Peptide T because, though they both show antiviral action, they have different mechanisms of action, which I will go into at length later on. Or combine AZT and ddC with Trental, which has been found to increase the effectiveness of AZT and ddC.

FDA DRUG TRIALS AND WHAT THEY MEAN TO YOU

There are three main steps in drug development and testing:

• *Phase 1 of clinical trials.* Researchers conduct trials on volunteers with the disease in question to learn whether the drug is safe for people to take. The trial is usually a dose-escalating study set up to test which doses become toxic in the human body and which are tolerated. In Phase 1 clinical trials, researchers raise the dosage until they find the largest amount of the drug that a person can take without toxicity.

• *Phase 2 of clinical trials.* A larger number of people are given the drug to see if it's safe to use and if it is efficacious—that is, if it works. Sometimes several hundred people are tested, and the trial can last from two months to two years. Recently, because of the limited number of medications available, the FDA has been approving drugs for HIV that have completed only Phase 2 of clinical trials.

• *Phase 3 of clinical trials.* Traditionally, however, a drug would have to complete a Phase 3 of clinical trials, which would test its long-term effects. Besides testing for long-term effects, researchers also look for rare side effects that may occur in only a few people after a long period. Drugs such as AZT, ddI, and ddC have all been approved in Phase 2 of trials, and the long-term effects are being tested now. Research is constantly being released on the long-term effects of these drugs. For example, in the beginning AZT was given at doses that varied from 300 to 500 mg. Not until two years had passed since approval was it proven that 500 mg is the most effective dose.

Traditionally, most drug trials were done with the actual substance being tested for effectiveness and a placebo as a "control." A placebo is a pill consisting of sugar or any other inert substance, and a placebo-controlled test compares the effects of the inert substance with those of the substance being tested. In these placebo-controlled trials, the recipient is not aware if he is getting the placebo or the actual drug. But in HIV trials this type of comparison has been frowned upon, because of the life-threatening nature of the infection. Therefore, many HIV trials are drug-comparison trials. Instead of comparing, say, ddI to a placebo, comparison trials might compare ddI with AZT. Such a trial would ask:

- Is ddI as effective as AZT?
- More effective?
- Are there better things about one or the other?

The only drug trials for HIV infection that are done with placebos are those for people with T cells above 500 who are at relatively low risk for developing opportunistic infections.

I hate to get into numbers and categories, but these distinctions are necessary in deciding when we are going to implement certain drugs and how to intercede. But remember, no matter what your numbers—whether they are considered "low" or "high"—*people are surviving all along the spectrum of HIV infection.* I will repeat this over and over again, because I don't want readers to fall into the better/worse trap: "I'm doing worse because my numbers are lower." No, you're *different,* not worse, and no matter what your levels, there's something you can do.

If you are considering volunteering to join a clinical trial, you would want to know

- which phase the trial is in;
- if the trial is a placebo-control trial;
- if you want to join a placebo-control trial;

- whether you qualify for the trial;
- what the conditions are for joining the trial; and
- whether the benefits outweigh the risks.

For instance, currently a Peptide T trial is going on in which participants are allowed to take AZT and are given Peptide T versus placebo. But the trial lasts for only three months, and after it is over everybody in the trial will be given Peptide T, by all early indications a very effective drug for neuropathy, and possibly an antiviral as well. So in this case, the trial might be very beneficial—volunteers will have a chance to be on a drug that people are paying exorbitant prices for on the black market or the underground drug trade, and you'll have a chance to be on high-quality, FDA-tested Peptide T for an unlimited time. In addition, allowing participants to take AZT offers another level of protection. Most trial participants are offered the tested drug long before it becomes generally available.

Often, drug trials have exclusionary criteria. Sometimes women are excluded because the drugs being tested could have an impact on childbearing or drug companies are afraid that women will become pregnant and drop out of the trial. Drug addicts are often excluded because of undependability. To decide whether you want to join a drug trial, you need to take all these factors into account. In the United States, an 800 telephone number exists for people to call to find out what drug trials are being run in your area: 1-800-TRIALS-A.

Personally, I recommend very few trials to my clients. Some of the substances I mention in this book are in trials, and where that is the case I offer my recommendations on whether or not the trial would be a good one to join. But I am comfortable about making this broad statement: I do not think HIV+ people should give up treatment that is currently working for a placebo-controlled trial. If you're on a substance and it's working for you—you're stabilized, your T cells are rising, things are going well—unless it is clear that the trial will yield more significant benefit than your current treatment, I would stick with what you're doing.

Drug trials are important, yes. But this is your life, and you must decide what's best for you. When faced with a drug trial that *might* work for you, it's difficult to weigh all the factors and decide whether or not to join. I hope the information provided here will help you decide.

CHAPTER 7

Acupuncture, Chiropractic, Chinese Medicine, and Homeopathy

Many people have decided to integrate these main complementary approaches into their treatment programs: acupuncture, chiropractic, Chinese medicine, and homeopathy. Each of these can have benefits—measurable benefits—in controlling the progression of HIV infection. I don't intend either to diminish or overstate the influence of any of these treatments on the progression of HIV infection. Instead, I want to urge you to treat these options scientifically—measure their efficacy in your particular case by looking for their effects in your regular bloodwork and on how you feel.

The point is, though these approaches are considered "alternative," their effects are quantifiable. In HIV treatment, these therapies are usually part of a larger program incorporating some drugs or natural interventions that have a track record with HIV infection. Therefore, these interventions can also be considered complementary to a mainstream medical treatment regimen. Care providers do not usually recommend these therapies alone, without other treatments, but some people choose on their own to use only these regimens to treat their HIV infection. However, you don't need to turn your back on science to use them; in fact, I have some doubts about using them alone in treating HIV progression. But you can *integrate* these treatments with more conventional ones and monitor the success of your choices by means of your laboratory reports.

The effects of the alternative and complementary options can be measured by bloodwork, but even more immediately they can be measured in terms of your sense of physical well-being, feelings of relaxation, and pain and tension reduction—all of the stresses that can have an effect on HIV infection. Some benefits are subjective, but that doesn't make them less real than numbers on a lab slip. After all, the point of the whole effort is to increase the feeling of well-being. Let's look to ourselves, not to our doctors or even our lab reports, to tell us how we feel!

Mark, whom I have worked with for more than five years, has integrated both acupuncture and chiropractic into his treatment regimen. In those five years, his bloodwork has remained stable at 695 T4 cells. He has used only natural interventions (to be discussed in Chapter 8) along with these therapies, and I certainly consider stabilization for five years a success.

Finally, let me make it clear that I'm not making miraculous claims for these approaches. I would be leery if someone told me that they had a cure for HIV infection. As far as I know, there are many effective treatments but no cures yet, although we can keep praying—and I do not think we should disregard the possibility that there will be a cure. Many of the complementary or alternative practitioners make a lot of claims about what they do. I prefer to choose practitioners who consider their therapies to be *helpful* in the holistic approach to your personal treatment plan and healing. So in choosing an acupuncturist or a chiropractor, I would recommend that you look for practitioners who feel that what they do is one facet of a complete plan rather than a cure for whatever ails you.

CONTROLLING ANXIETY

Over the last two decades, many Americans have been drawn to the healing arts of other cultures and have found ways to incorporate these approaches into their lives. Acupuncture, chiropractic, and Chinese medicine all have significant stress-reducing capabilities, as hundreds of thousands of people have learned to their great benefit. But there are still those people who brush aside these holistic approaches as "New Age psychobabble." If you share this negative impression, I want to pause for a second and speak to you directly. Mainly, I want to ask you to take another look at these options in the context of HIV infection.

I have seen many of my patients—even some of the most hardened, cynical, streetwise city people—come to the realization that alternative therapies such as those described in this chapter not only make sense but answer a need that no conventional treatment addresses. That need is for anxiety control—a way to calm and endure the fear that is an inevitable result of living with a *potentially* life-threatening dis-ease. Western medicine is notoriously disease-centered, leaving patients to struggle along with the emotional consequences as best they can, and this is where stress-reduction techniques that have served in other cultures for centuries can be of inestimable value.

You've read the stories; I don't need to provide you with testimonials. Without attempting to convince you by citing a million anecdotes, if you have shied away from these "softer" approaches, I urge and encourage you to take another look. More than one patient has told me, "I can deal with the physical problems of HIV infection—I deal with them as they arise, one at a time. It's the anxiety that I can't handle. I'm scared all the time and it's ruining my life." If this sounds familiar, and if you long ago turned your back on these approaches to healing, you may well find that the very problems your care providers never address are the ones that holistic healing arts deal with most effectively of all.

Personally, I have had positive experiences with most of these approaches. Acupuncture gave me my energy back and I was able to function again after a long period of chronic fatigue, while chiropractic relieved my chronic lower-back pain. And I often rely on Chinese herbs for fending off day-to-day colds and infections.

ACUPUNCTURE

Acupuncture is an ancient traditional Chinese medical technique that stimulates the natural flow of energy within the body. The theories of acupuncture are based on the belief that the human body has the built-in power to heal itself. The practice of acupuncture is meant to stimulate and release that natural power.

Either to maintain health or prevent disease by restoring the body's natural balance, the acupuncturist inserts threadlike needles through the skin at specific points in the body. My personal experience has been that acupuncture is almost completely painless. On the occasions when I did feel pain at the insertion of a needle, my acupuncturist explained, "That is where the energy is blocked from flowing through your body." If you breathe deeply during an acupuncture treatment, any pain you might feel will subside very quickly, and you are likely to feel a positive surge of energy. Lying on an acupuncture table, I have actually felt the flow of energy increase throughout my body after the insertion of the needles.

Different acupuncture points are related to different physical conditions. One approved use of acupuncture in the United States is for drug withdrawal. The acupuncture helps relax the patient to the point where some of the withdrawal symptoms subside and the person's urgent motivation to use drugs decreases. This technique has been proven effective and is covered by most insurance companies. Many insurance companies cover acupuncture treatments for other conditions as well.

Some of the most beneficial effects of acupuncture are the relief of:

- high blood pressure
- sleepless nights
- headaches
- stress
- digestive problems
- the pain of peripheral neuropathy
- the side effects from drugs prescribed for HIV

My acupuncturist has had enormous success in relieving peripheral neuropathy, which is very common in HIV infection, usually in the legs or hands as a pain or tingling, almost like an arthritic feeling.

In choosing an acupuncturist, ask your support group of HIV+ people or your local HIV community-based organization, which the Resource Guide will help you find, for a referral to someone who has been working with HIV+ patients.

Most acupuncturists use disposable needles. However, some acupuncturists do clean and reuse their needles, and this is not the type of treatment you want. Make sure the acupuncturist you choose uses disposable needles and discards all needles after each session.

Choosing acupuncture as a complementary treatment is a wonderful idea, but in seeking out your acupuncturist I'd recommend speaking to HIV+ patients of specific practitioners to see if they are getting results.

As for availability and insurance coverage, by now acupuncture has earned a place in even the most conservative institutions. It is often available at public clinics where Medicaid is accepted, and many private insurance carriers cover it as well. Still, try to choose an M.D. (medical doctor) who does acupuncture, since insurance companies tend to reimburse these practitioners more readily than they do others. Take these factors into account when you are shopping around for an acupuncturist. If you have insurance, try to find an acupuncturist who accepts your plan.

As a complementary therapy, one acupuncture treatment every week or every other week is definitely beneficial to the healing process where HIV infection is concerned. But if your T4 cells are below 300, you might choose two sessions per week for additional benefit. Although Western medicine has not completely recognized acupuncture, this practice is helping thousands of HIV+ patients, and the combination of Western medicine and acupuncture is a very powerful healing regimen.

Among the studies presented at the Eighth International AIDS Conference, one chronicled the results of HIV+s using acupuncture, reporting an extended survival rate and a substantial reduction in symptoms and side effects to HIV-related drugs (PoB 3393). Other benefits cited were the frequent normalization of CBC (complete blood counts); reduction in fatigue, abnormal sweating, diarrhea, and acute skin rashes; and, in some patients, a 15- to 20-pound weight gain. These benefits cannot be minimized; nevertheless, Western practitioners often do dismiss or diminish them.

In fact, many Western doctors often try to write off acupuncture and other Chinese medical practices as quackery. Such an attitude can undermine the effectiveness of these complementary treatments. But you must be guided by how you feel and what your bloodwork tells you. Remember, if you walk into an acupuncture treatment feeling totally stressed and you get up off that table feeling released, relieved, relaxed, without tension, that is definite benefit. Trust your heart and ask yourself:

- Are my symptoms getting better?
- How do I really feel?

One final note: acupuncture has been proven to affect the blood level of neuropeptides, the body's "communicators" that send messages to various body systems to increase their action. No matter what intervention you choose, your belief will be a factor in its effectiveness. Remember: this practice is thousands of years old, and benefits have been demonstrated for much longer than the history of Western medical science. I consider acupuncture, of all the bodywork interventions, to be the most beneficial for the HIV+ person.

CHIROPRACTIC

Chiropractic and acupuncture are related to each other in theory. Both are concerned with dismantling blockages to optimum human functioning. Chiropractic concerns itself with structural blocks in the spinal column called subluxations. These blockages occur where vertebrae crowd the nerves, reducing their ability to supply the correct messages to other organs and tissues. To rid the body of these blockages, the chiropractor manipulates the spinal column, allowing all the nerves to function fully and supply all the proper messages between other organs, the brain, and tissue. In theory, freeing these impulses gives the body its optimum healing power.

Certainly chiropractic can relieve back pain, and a good adjustment—the term used to describe a chiropractic session—can significantly reduce stress, headaches, and tension. People often complain that this relief is temporary, but I answer by pointing out that the effects of pills are temporary, too—when the effects of one begin to fade, you take another. And having an adjustment, as compared to putting something unnatural into your body, seems to me a much less toxic and less invasive approach to healing.

Again, chiropractic adjustments on a weekly basis are an

excellent complementary therapy for people with HIV infection. I'm not recommending that people do chiropractic, Chinese medicine, acupuncture, homeopathy, and maybe ten other therapies. As I stated earlier, the point is to combine a few different treatments to formulate a treatment plan that you feel comfortable with and that, once you've implemented it, gives you some measurable benefit, both in your bloodwork and in how you feel. Try them all, then choose one, two, or three that give you the most benefit.

There are many types of chiropractic adjustments:

• the standard adjustment, in which the spinal column is manipulated and aligned;
• nonforce practices, utilizing reflexology. In this practice, the bottom of the foot is treated as a reflection of the body as a whole and is tested to reveal specific trouble spots. In accordance with the results of this test, the chiropractor moves specific bones, relieving subluxations and therefore promoting healing;
• other types of chiropractic practices. These vary according to practitioners and different theories of chiropractic manipulation.

Any type of chiropractic adjustment that seems to work for you—and that is a personal decision—would be a perfect complementary addition to your holistic regimen. If you are comfortable with the practitioner, if you feel a difference in your health—less tension, less back pain, more energy after the treatments—then trust your body's messages and stick with that person.

As with acupuncture, I would try to pick a chiropractor who has some experience with HIV+ people, who has been recommended by your community-based HIV organization, and who accepts your insurance.

Chiropractic might be most useful for structural problems, the constant pain of which can affect your emotional and physical well-being. In my own case, my right hip is misaligned, which causes constant low-level pain. During periods when that pain is most unrelenting, I develop more colds, flus, and allergies and my energy diminishes and irritability level rises. With consistent chiropractic adjustments—once a month to every two weeks—the hip stays in place and the other effects disappear.

Structural imbalance can result in association with other symptoms of HIV infection. Ron, a patient with HIV infection, developed shingles—also known as herpes zoster—after he was in a car accident and sustained a whiplash. His neck was under constant stress, and the manifestation of the herpes zoster was the eventual result. He began to have regular chiropractic adjustments to treat his neck—since the problem was so serious he began at three times a week for a month—and the herpes zoster began clearing up. After the first week, Ron also began to use Zovirax, which is the Western treatment of choice for shingles. The relief of his neck pain sparked the healing of the shingles, and in a record two weeks the shingles were gone. Zovirax, by the way, is not known to provide relief so quickly on its own.

To summarize, chiropractic is useful as adjunct therapy—therapy used to support other treatments—but where structural problems exist it is central to the body's healing process. It is also highly beneficial as stress reduction—I know of one practitioner who provides a chiropractic adjustment and acupuncture in one appointment, an ideal combination.

MASSAGE

Massage is one of the best techniques for stress reduction. There are many different types of massage, including shiatsu, Swedish, and reflexology. It might take several visits to different practitioners to find one that you are comfortable with. In New York and Los Angeles, the Centers for Living (see Resource Guide) provide free massage for HIV+ people. If you can't afford a professional massage, ask a friend or lover to accommodate you.

For HIV in general, acupuncture, chiropractic, and massage are all good adjunct therapies. I would try all three, choosing one for regular weekly treatments and the others as adjunct therapies, possibly one time a month.

CHINESE HERBOLOGY

Like acupuncture, Chinese herbology has been around for thousands of years. Many HIV+ people have chosen Chinese herbal therapies for HIV infection because of their low toxicity and possible benefits. Research conducted in China has shown that certain ingredients in Chinese herbs can restore immune functions. Unfortunately, not much documentation exists about Chinese herbs and their positive effects. Again, monitoring your own bloodwork is absolutely essential when using a Chinese herbal intervention.

All herbs are plants. Many plants are not medicinal herbs, though many common weeds are highly beneficial. The fleshy plants that die each year are commonly considered herbs, and pharmaceutical companies have discovered some of their most useful medicines in plants.

Although some herbs have been singled out, it is difficult to point out one or two herbs and say these are the herbs to take and these are the ones that would be most helpful in HIV infection. If you are interested in pursuing this course, I recommend that you seek out a Chinese herbologist with some experience in HIV infection to put together an herbal regimen for your use. Many acupuncturists use herbs along with their treatments.

Certain herbs have been put together and sold as herbal formulas. Two—Composition A and Enhance—are used very commonly in HIV infection, and I will discuss them in Chapter 8 when I detail specific natural interventions. To learn about individual herbs that have proven useful in HIV treatment and their possible benefits, you'll need to research further. I've listed the more common Chinese herbs and herbal preparations used with HIV at the end of this section, and you'll find some book titles in the Resource Guide for additional reading. However, neither is an exhaustive list, and again I recommend working with a practicing Chinese herbalist.

If you have a Chinatown or a Chinese practitioner in your community, you'll find the herbs inexpensive and easily available. And if you and your practitioner put together a regimen combining herbs, in most cases you need not be concerned about over-medicating yourself. Owing to the herbs' low toxicity, most people experience no adverse side effects from them.

When practitioners create an herbal regimen, most are concerned with the balance of *yin* and *yang*. Most HIV+ patients show symptoms and signs of deficiency in both yin and yang. These deficiencies usually involve the kidneys, spleen, and lungs.

Yin deficiency symptoms usually include sensations of heat and flushing, sensations of thirst and dry throat, and, common in HIV, night sweats. Yang deficiency symptoms can include sensations of chilliness, e.g., cold extremities, dependent edema (swelling of the legs), frequent urination, colorless urine, and loose stools.

The practitioner seeks to balance the yin and yang of the patient. Chinese medicine and herbal remedies should help to strengthen the areas which are involved in these deficiencies (usually in the lungs, spleen, and kidneys).

For yin deficiencies, herbs that produce heat (e.g., some types of ginseng) are not recommended. When working with an herbalist, inquire as to whether you are yin- or yang-deficient. Most but not all HIV+s are yin-deficient and should therefore remain cautious with herbs that create heat in the body.

Some people develop a detoxifying effect. This detoxification is very common in response to the more natural interventions. When the herbs are put into the body, toxins are pushed out, and the movement of these toxins elicits certain reactions, sometimes skin rashes or fevers. Most practitioners would say, "Just go through this period until the reaction stops." Some would advise you to reduce the amount of herbs you are taking to make the detoxifying period less intense. I make this point about detoxifying not to scare you but to illustrate that the process is actually very healthful. The response is palpable evidence that the body is being relieved of the toxins it takes in on a daily basis. The only problem with the fever and flu-like symptoms of detoxification is their similarity to the symptoms of many OIs. The easiest way to be confident that these symptoms are benign and unrelated to an OI is to stop the herbal regimen, thus ending the detox and symptoms.

Echinacea is one of the most commonly used herbal preparations for immune modulation. Most documentation on herbs cites this plant as a potent immune stimulator. Echinacea is usually in a tincture that has been used by many herbologists to stimulate the immune system to help with colds, flus, and other common illnesses. One researcher—Lawrence E. Badgly, M.D., author of

Healing AIDS Naturally—reported on one HIV patient with a starting T_4/T_8 ratio (also referred to as CD_4/CD_8 ratio) of .35 and an absolute T_4 number of 299. After 30 drops of echinacea three times daily for three weeks, the ratio went up to .50 and the absolute T_4-cell count went up to 349.

Now, this was a report on only one patient and the information was not complete on what other treatments this person might be combining with the echinacea. And it's important to remember that, especially with HIV infection, different things seem to work in different people. But when you're talking about relatively nontoxic interventions and you're in the higher range of T cells, the possibility exists that these therapies will stop the progression of HIV infection before you have to get the very toxic medications. Echinacea is one of the more widely used immune modulators, and evidence of its efficacy is greater than with herbs that are used less frequently, but 30 drops three times a day is a large amount and can be quite pricey. Other alternatives might give you more benefit for your money.

Most commonly, Chinese herbs are combined and cooked to make either a soup or a tea, or powdered forms can be taken as pills. Because cooking the herbs is time-consuming and produces a tea with an unpleasant smell and taste, most people prefer using the pills or tablets.

In this book I deal mainly with medical interventions, so this section on herbs and the other alternative interventions is intended as an overview, useful when you do your own research. There are many different herbal preparations. Besides Chinese herbs, Egyptian, Greek, Roman, and contemporary herbs of many types are available from herbologists and herb stores. If you decide to go this route, you'll need to find your own way to an herbal regimen that suits you personally. Books on herbs and HIV are available; use the Resource Guide to point you in the right direction. Once again, I strongly suggest that you consult a practitioner if you are considering putting together an herbal preparation.

CHINESE HERBS USED WITH HIV INFECTION

Agrimonia	Ephedra	Millettia
Alisma	Eugenia	Peony
Artemisia	Forsythia	Polygonum
apiacea	Gandoderma	Preparatum et recens
Astragalus	Gardenia	rehmannia
Atractylodes alba	Glycyrrhiza	Prunella
Cinnamon	radix	Salvia
Codonopsis	Grifola	Schizandra
Coix	Isatis folium	Scrophularia zingiber
Cornus	Lily	sicca
Deer antler	Lithospermum	Tricosanthes radix
Dioscorea	Lonicera	Tricosanthes semen
Echinacea	Lycium cortex	Viola

HERBAL PREPARATIONS

Composition A
Composition
Clear Heat
Enhance

HOMEOPATHY

Homeopathy is a practice that was first developed in Germany in the 1800s. Practitioners found that different herbs and minerals caused symptoms that were identical to the symptoms of each of the diseases known to humankind. The first homeopaths administered infinitesimal amounts of these herbs and minerals to induce symptoms of the disease under treatment. In response, the patient's body would build up a natural immunity to the disease. The reasoning is similar to that behind the vaccine principle: you give a small amount of a certain virus to stimulate a natural immune response to that virus. Homeopathy has been in use ever since.

One major point: *Homeopathy must be done with a homeopathic practitioner. Do not practice homeopathic methods on your own.*

Homeopathy has become very popular with HIV+ people,

and many are claiming huge positive results. If your T cells are above 700, or even above 500, you really have the opportunity to pick and choose among different remedies to see if they work for you. Even if T4 cells are below 500, these remedies could show benefit, but I would not recommend them alone. Follow your lab results. They are your key.

IN SUMMARY

All four of the major approaches described here interact very well with Western medical procedures. Most of the herbs and all of the acupuncture, chiropractic, and homeopathic treatments can be integrated with each other and with most Western treatments without any negative effects. Of course, it's absolutely imperative that you check with your practitioners, both Western and complementary, to make sure that the specific substances you are taking do not interact in possibly harmful ways, but it has been my experience that acupuncture, chiropractic and massage can be combined with *any* treatment regimen whatsoever. Also, some practitioners say, "You can do those things, but they don't work." If there is substantial proof of this, okay, but most of the time this statement is made out of fear and ignorance. Check with your practitioner for homeopathic treatments that combine well with Western medicine.

BREAKING THE MYTHS

Myth: Alternative therapies are for flakes, airheads, and "New Age" types who turn away from traditional approaches, and they have no benefit whatsoever.
Truth: The main benefit of taking control of your medical treatment is the freedom this gives you to draw from *every* type of treatment, from highly conventional to alternative, depending on your medical situation, your knowledge of alternatives, and your temperament. Many alternative practices have good evidence of *some* benefit in treatment of HIV infection.

Myth: Herbs and homeopathic remedies cannot be taken with other medications.

Truth: As we established earlier, check with your practitioner. Most herbs and homeopathic remedies work well with other medications. In addition, check with herbologists for preparations that can reduce the toxicity and side effects of some Western therapies.

Myth: Herbs are not strong enough to fight HIV infection. **Truth:** When your T4 cells are above 400, herbs can be of great benefit before you try the more aggressive/toxic Western therapies. When your T4 cells are below 400, herbs can help reduce toxicity and side effects while adding support to the body's healing systems.

CHAPTER 8

Natural Interventions

In July 1992, I attended the Eighth International AIDS Conference in Amsterdam. The published report of the conference contained more than 3,000 abstracts—reports of small studies that test the effectiveness of treatment interventions. Of those abstracts published in the report, only fourteen listed in the report's index focused on alternative therapies (including the natural interventions to be discussed in this chapter).

In this clear emphasis on mainstream intervention, someone, I'm not sure who, is making a grave mistake. Is it the government, which has so inflated the cost of the drug-approval process that a treatment has to be backed by a major drug company to stand a chance? Or is it the conservative streak in the medical establishment, which has demanded so much evidence of the most benign substances to substantiate treatment efficacy that vitamins and inexpensive substances become a "business loss" to test? Whoever carries the blame, it is simply infuriating to see new evidence of a system fueled and diverted by greed while lives are being lost.

One of the more memorable events at the 1992 conference was when the group ACT UP, the AIDS Coalition to Unleash Power, staged what they called an "action." This action consisted of entering the conference floor and tearing down the exhibition booth of Astra, a wealthy American drug company. ACT UP took this particular action to draw attention to the fact that Astra is charging $30,000 a year for the drug foscarnet, an antiviral approved for the treatment of CMV. ACT UP claims that the company could charge $10,000 and *still* make a hefty profit on foscarnet. Astra argues that it could not recoup its investment at that price. Something is certainly very wrong when a company must charge more than most people's annual salary for a life-extending drug.

Although many medical doctors discount the effectiveness of alternative therapies, one of the abstracts accepted for the Amsterdam conference sums up my own feelings about alternatives. It stated that substances that are widely available and inexpensive have shown a degree of efficacy in the treatment of HIV. It went on to say that "preliminary research results can identify possible treatments of HIV, which can then be screened by individuals in real-life situations, thereby providing information about usefulness of treatments long before formal research is complete" (PoB 3391).

That's exactly what I'm saying here. Let's allow HIV+ people access to the information available on alternative treatments, even if it is limited, to decide if *they* would like to use those drugs. Then they and their care providers can monitor their bloodwork to determine whether the therapies they have chosen are effective in their particular cases.

The quote from the abstract, by David Baker, R.N., M.S.N., an HIV specialist, continues:

- "Anecdotal reports are an untapped resource."
- "Specific treatments benefit some people, but not all."
- "People with HIV tend to maintain their health better when they are informed about, involved in, and choosing their own treatment program."

The abstract went on to name the six key factors that go into deciding on an alternative, all six of which are completely consistent with the philosophy of treatments and patient participation detailed in this book, the same comments I have been making for the past five years.

1. Check lab test trends.
2. Weigh possible benefits versus possible side effects.
3. Intuition, which meditation can clarify.
4. Willingness to endure side effects.

5. Willingness to take risk.
6. Desire to live.

There is a serious need for Western medicine to recognize approaches to medicine in cultures that differ from its own. Herbal remedies, acupuncture, and healing from the earth are practices that are much older than Western medicine. They all have their uses, proven over the centuries, and it is just plain arrogant to ignore this body of knowledge.

If you stop and think about it, what do our medical policy-makers have to be arrogant about? No one can argue with the fact that our health-care system is deteriorating. It's difficult to ignore the headlines. Still, it's possible to view this breakdown as a *positive* development, in that it might open our medical practices and permit the merging of many medical cultures, which would make it more universal.

But you don't have to wait; you can do the merging on your own. All you need is the willingness to study. Get the facts, and you will be able to make your own educated decisions.

Some argue that reading, reading, reading in an all-out search for relevant information is a way of obsessing on HIV infection. But in my view, obsessing on your condition means running in little mental circles without breaking out and collecting the relevant information and taking action, using the information you have researched. Studying, on the other hand, is empowerment:

- You study.
- You make a decision.
- And then you move on, knowing that you are powerless over the results.
- Still, though you come to terms with all possibilities, you *believe* in the positive.

MAKING THE DECISION

Believe me, I am not making light of the decision-making process. I have watched enough people wrestle with treatment choices to know that many factors are involved. But you can make things easier on yourself by avoiding common pitfalls and staying with the evidence.

For example, many people lose their ability to advocate for themselves because of reluctance to disagree with their physicians. They are still holding on to the old idea that doctors are healers and that if they don't have the answers, then nobody does. Others have codependent tendencies that do not allow them to go against their physicians' advice.

But listen: this is *your* life. *You* must make the decisions. Don't put your life in someone else's hands who may have less information than what you're reading right here in this book. There is nothing wrong with doctors, but there *is* something wrong with our system when, even though you travel to a conference, you have to use a magnifying glass to read 3,000+ abstracts to get the latest information about AIDS.

Most people, including doctors, lack the time to sift through a report of that size, so they remain ignorant of the full range of possibilities in HIV treatment. Drawing attention to those possibilities and to the many resources available were major motivations for me in writing this book. In the Resource Guide, I have listed those resources and explained how you can get hold of them. The same resources available to your doctor are right out there available to you.

Remember, the turning point in a treatment decision could be how toxicity weighs out against possible benefit—and most natural treatments usually have no toxicity whatsoever. One of my colleagues once called such treatments the "what-the-hell" drugs.

As to the benefits, they may be measurable, but there isn't enough money available to research these options the way the FDA wants them researched. Still, some empirical evidence does exist that the alternative treatments I describe in this chapter yield benefits to some HIV+ people. And then there are anecdotal reports—also referred to in the Amsterdam abstract—in which individual people testify to the effectiveness of alternative treatments.

Finally, while it is clear that *some* treatments work on *some* people, not all treatments work on everybody—not even AZT works on everyone. That is why you need to know how to read your own bloodwork, the ultimate measurement of a treatment's effectiveness.

Remember the treatment categories: antivirals, immune modulators, treatments for opportunistic infections, and prophylaxes for opportunistic infections (OIs). These four categories apply to alternative as well as mainstream treatments, although some alternatives, like some mainstream drugs, have dual capabilities. It is not uncommon to choose an alternative to back up a Western medical choice—for example, taking a detoxifying herbal regimen if you are on AZT or other natural interventions that can reduce the side effects of toxic drugs. Another common example for those taking Bactrim (discussed in Chapter 14) three times a week as a PCP prophylaxis is to take acidophilus—a natural substance to replace the flora in the stomach that Bactrim eliminates.

So, on we go, into the alternatives, working with the evidence and making decisions for ourselves.

SUPER BLUE-GREEN ALGAE (BLUE-GREEN ALGAE)

Science News, The New York Times (Washington Talk section), and even the mainstream book *AIDS Therapies* have all reported benefits of algae in HIV infection. *Science News* (August 26, 1989) stated, "Compounds found in two strains of blue-green algae

---

Brand Versus Drug Names

As I mentioned earlier, in discussing specific treatments I identify products both by brand name and the name of the substance the drug is made from (sometimes called the "generic" name). Sometimes the differences between these two are quite subtle—for example, Super Blue-Green Algae is the company Cell Tech's brand name for the substance blue-green algae. But some brand names, especially of pharmaceutical substances, are completely different from the generic term. For example, Trental, a product made by Hoechst-Roussel Pharmaceuticals, Inc., is made from the substance pentoxifylline.

In the treatment descriptions, I cite brand name first, with generic drug name in parentheses. Where there is no specific brand, the single name given is the drug substance. Sometimes, a specific brand from a particular company must be used; in such cases I specify this in the description.

protect human T cells from destruction by the AIDS virus, HIV. The findings are very preliminary. . . ."

These articles were all based on a study (published in the June 2, 1989, issue of the *Journal of the National Cancer Institute*) titled "AIDS Antiviral Sulfolipids from Cyanobacteria (Blue-Green Algae)," which showed that, in laboratory petri dishes, ingredients in algae protected T cells from the attack of HIV. As you probably know, what happens in petri dishes (called *in vitro* research) is often not the same as what happens in the body (*in vivo*). As a matter of fact, one recent article stated that this benefit would probably require very high amounts of blue-green algae. But algae contains so many vitamins, amino acids, and trace minerals that it probably cannot fail to be beneficial for many other reasons besides interfering with HIV directly. Most nutritionists agree. The nutrition specialist Lark Lands, Ph.D., has stated that HIV+ people have deficiencies of nutrients that begin very early and can affect HIV progression. Blue-green algae has a well balanced, easily digested nutritional profile.

Since no major drug company owns the world's reserves of blue-green algae from which they could profit, the research is slow. Super Blue-Green Algae, made by Cell Tech, is the brand used most often in HIV+s who choose to explore this remedy because of its superior quality, freeze-drying capability, and reliable freshness. At a recent lecture I gave, two blue-green algae takers stood up and related their personal experiences. Both told of rises in the T_4 cells—one of 200 points and one of 300 points. I have seen one patient's T_4 cells go from 695 to 1,200 during the period in which he took blue-green algae, B_{12}, and Vitamin C. Owing to the scarcity of research on this treatment, it is necessary for us to pay attention to such anecdotal reports.

As with all treatments, although blue-green algae has benefited some people, it may not help others. Still, because it is a nontoxic therapy, I usually recommend blue-green algae as the basis for most treatment regimens.

Algae contains an amino acid profile and a host of trace minerals that not only may benefit HIV+ people but have other positive effects as well. One of the most common, reported by both people who are HIV+ and people who are not, is a feeling of increased energy. A broad spectrum of users swear by the energy-boosting effects of blue-green algae.

Finally, much of the literature on natural therapy, including

Dr. Lark Lands's report, "Therapeutic Basics for People Living with HIV," states that the algae stimulates the thymus gland. The thymus is responsible for maturing T4 cells and supporting the immune system.

The benefits of blue-green algae are multifaceted. Since HIV progression has been so definitely linked to vitamin and mineral deficiencies, a vitamin supplement is essential. Using a regular "one-a-day" type vitamin is okay, but many of the chemically formulated vitamins go undigested, and are eliminated by the body. You will notice a dark color to your urine at those times. A better supplement is a "food source" vitamin, made from a con-centrated food or foods that provide the vitamin and mineral supplementation. This type of supplement is absorbed better and is therefore much more efficient. Ninety percent of most "food source" vitamins are made from blue-green algae. I usually use the algae directly; it provides a full range of amino acids, which make proteins, which in turn make the cells of the body. Algae also contains chlorophyll, which helps build blood cells, and high levels of vitamin B_{12} and beta-carotene.

Freeze-dried algae supplements are most beneficial, since this process does not kill the active enzymes that make the algae so nutritious. When freeze-dried products remain on store shelves for more than six months, potency can be lost. For this reason I suggest ordering directly from the company; it's cheaper, too.

There are reports of people taking too much algae too soon and developing pimples or skin rashes. This is the detox response common with natural medicines that I mentioned in Chapter 7. You can easily avoid this reaction by starting with low doses and building up. There does not seem to be any other toxicity related to blue-green algae.

Algae comes in capsules and powder. The powder can be mixed in juice or water.

Resource: No prescription is needed. For information on a slow-start program, dosage, and ordering, call Nick Siano's of-fice, listed in the Resource Guide.

VITAMIN C THERAPY

Many holistic magazines, and some mainstream ones too, have reported on the benefits to HIV+ people of high-dose vitamin C.

There was even an abstract submitted at the Amsterdam conference on the benefits of this therapy (PoB 3697). All these articles and the abstract were based on a study done at the Linus Pauling Institute by Steve Harakeh and his colleagues. The abstract of the study stated, "In chronically infected cells expressing HIV at peak levels, ascorbate [vitamin C] reduced the levels of extracellular reverse transcriptase (RT) activity by greater than 99 percent and of P24 antigen by 90 percent in the culture supernatant." Reverse transcriptase is the enzyme which helps HIV replicate, and P24 antigen is the viral protein; reducing these levels would suggest reducing HIV activity.

This one study has been the basis for many, many prescriptions by naturalists of high doses of vitamin C and in many cases intravenous vitamin C therapy for people who are HIV+. Anecdotal reports are mixed. Some people seem to get benefit and some do not, but that is probably the case with all therapies.

For a long time, many mainstream medical professionals claimed that high-dose vitamin C would induce kidney stones, since it lowers copper, calcium, manganese, magnesium, and B_{12} in the body. This and other theories have not been borne out—I have found no reports of an association between kidney stones and high-dose vitamin C in any of the medical literature, nor do anecdotal reports support this theory. Nevertheless, most naturalists believe that it is important to take a supplement to increase the minerals depleted by vitamin C. Blue-green algae contains all of these trace minerals, and would serve this purpose well.

The dosage recommended by the Harakeh study was a minimum of 10,000 milligrams (mg) per day. The activity of one type of vitamin C, called ester C, available from many different companies (one brand of ester C is manufactured by Natrol) is assimilated by the body at four times the milligram level on the bottle. This means that taking 500 mg of ester C gives you 2,000 mg of vitamin C activity, and there is no need to take doses larger than the activity level. Five ester Cs daily amount to 10,000 mg of vitamin C activity.

However, Michelle Alpert, D.O., a New York doctor who is an expert in vitamin therapy, considers the 500-mg ester C dosage insufficient. She states that ester C does not contain "free radical scavengers," which are found in normal ascorbate (vitamin C). Free radicals are elements in the blood that can contribute to viral and/or cancerous growths. She recommends a mixture of ester C and regular ascorbate as the best vitamin C regimen for HIV infection. She also regularly prescribes vitamin C drips. These are the recommendations I have adopted.

Another prominent New York doctor, Bernard Bihari, believes that people with fewer than 300 T cells might not benefit from high-dose vitamin C. He states that the level of alpha interferon (one of the body's natural antiviral proteins) in people with fewer than 300 T cells is already too high and points out that vitamin C produces additional alpha interferon, thus exacerbating HIV rather than reducing its effects. This effect is also noted in an article by Marcus Boon in *PWA Newsline* (August 1992, Issue 79). The article states that vitamin C "apparently increases alpha-interferon levels—which again are associated with increased likelihood of progression to AIDS."

With all this controversy, you'll need to pay close attention to your bloodwork to decide whether or not to pursue this treatment. But by combining all the recommendations, it's possible to come up with some guidelines on high-dose vitamin C as a treatment for HIV infection:

• This treatment is not recommended for people with T4-cell counts below 300. It is at this point that high alpha interferon levels are suspected.
• For people above 300, I recommend combining the ester C with regular ascorbate (vitamin C) until the 10,000-mg dose is achieved—that is, 2 ester C ($500 \times 2 = 1,000 \times 4 = 4,000$) with 6,000 mg of regular ascorbate. The entire dose of C must be split up and taken in equal intervals throughout the day. Vitamin C is water soluble and is quickly digested by the body and turned into urine. Both types of vitamin C are available without a prescription in pill or powdered form.

In addition, both the articles and the conference abstract suggest that vitamin C might enhance the action of another natural therapy, called NAC (discussed in the next section), which might have some antiviral effect. For the person with more than 300 T4 cells, these two therapies together are a viable option. When T4 cells are below 300, I sometimes recommend a total of 3,000 mg of vitamin C a day to help protect against common colds. The smaller amounts of vitamin C do not seem to have any negative effect.

Note that vitamin C seems to be associated with what vitamin experts call "bowel tolerance" (diarrhea develops when the saturation of vitamin C has been reached). So, if you decide on this therapy, you must build slowly, starting with one pill—one ester C 500 or 2,000 mg ascorbate per day—and adding one pill every other day until you have a soft bowel movement. At that point, return to the last dose, stay there for at least a week, maybe two, and then, if you have not reached the recommended dosage, continue the gradual increase.

Buyers Clubs

In the early eighties HIV+ people were extremely frustrated by the lack of treatment options available for HIV infection. A group of HIV+ people joined together to form what would later be called a buyers club.

This original group had read about the possible benefit of an egg lipid formula called AL 721, not yet available in the U.S. but available in Israel. The group decided to purchase the product, ship it in, and sell it to HIV+ people interested in exploring this option. Toxicity and side effects were taken into account, and since they were virtually nonexistent, the group decided the benefits of the product outweighed any risks. Years later AL 721 was proved useless in treating HIV though many reported having benefited from the treatment.

The group decided to import other experimental treatments, making them available to the HIV community. At first there were concerns that the FDA would not allow them to continue. But it seemed they were operating under a loophole in the law which allowed people with life-threatening illnesses to import medications from other countries for their personal use.

The group flourished and similar buyers clubs sprang up all over the country. Today almost every large city has a buyers club for HIV+ people, importing drugs that are not yet FDA approved in the U.S. or importing FDA-approved drugs from other countries where they are half the price. You will need a prescription for any FDA-approved drug you wish to purchase from a buyers club; in addition, you may need a prescription for certain non−FDA-approved drugs. Individual buyers clubs will provide prescription guidelines.

You will find a list of buyers clubs in the Resource Guide. Contacting your local buyers club for a brochure of available products would be beneficial in your gathering of information.

Some people never develop diarrhea from vitamin C. If you already have diarrhea, it's important to wait until the condition resolves before investigating this treatment option.

Resource: Your local health-food store.

SOLGAR NAC (N-ACETYL CYSTEINE)

NAC is an amino acid derivative approved in other countries for bronchitis treatment and Tylenol overdoses. It is available in the United States without a prescription. NAC has been observed to lower circulating levels of TNF (tumor necrosis factor), which can increase HIV replication and cause wasting syndrome. In addition, NAC seems to raise the level of the enzyme glutathione, which is lowered in people with HIV infection. Decreased glutathione levels, which HIV can cause, are known to make cells vulnerable to apoptosis, a function of the body that eliminates old cells. Decreases in glutathione can cause apoptosis to dysfunction and eliminate necessary T4 cells. Luc Montagnier, discoverer of HIV, has studied fifteen patients on 600–1,200 mg daily of NAC for six months and found that after this treatment T4 cells no longer underwent dysfunctional apoptosis, probably because NAC increases the level of circulating glutathione. In addition, the decrease in circulating TNF and the rise in glutathione levels seem to be related to HIV exacerbation and, in some way, to wasting syndrome and food absorption. Some practitioners have tried prescribing glutathione supplements to alleviate this problem, but these supplements are not absorbed properly and do not raise glutathione levels as NAC does.

NAC is a variant of an amino acid called cysteine. The European versions are sold in buyers clubs and the amino acid derivative is available at most health-food stores. Different vitamin manufacturers make NAC, or N-acetyl cysteine; the most popular brand seems to be Solgar's NAC.

One study on the use of NAC presented at the Eighth International AIDS Conference (PoB 3013) chronicled lowered P24 antigen levels, which suggests lowered viral activity. But, as I explained in Chapter 5, the meaning of the P24 antigen test is not fully understood. Other articles, in *AIDS Treatment News* and *Outweek,* also discuss the possibility of NAC's benefits. Most recently, an article in PWA Health Group's *Notes from the Under-*

ground suggests that food-absorption problems (see below for more on absorption), which were noted in *AIDS Treatment News,* were related to disease progression.

There is some question as to whether NAC is absorbed properly through the stomach, and whether the body will maintain a blood level of the substance high enough to permit it to be effective. The absorption problems associated with NAC might be related to the very condition this treatment is intended to reverse by lowering TNF and raising glutathione. As stated earlier, with these levels out of range, food-absorption efficiency is decreased. Absorption of drugs and supplements may be hindered too. As I'll discuss in Chapter 10, Trental, a circulatory drug, has also been found to decrease TNF levels. When TNF levels are high, laboratory studies show an almost completely reversed anti-retroviral effect of AZT or ddC as well as increases in the replication of HIV and wasting syndrome.

If high circulating TNF levels somehow reverse the effect of AZT and ddC, and also interfere with absorption, those two

---

Absorption

Throughout this book the issue of "absorption" comes up several times. In recent research and in doctors' opinions, absorption of nutrients from food, of treatment intervention drugs, of supplements, and of any other product introduced into the body through the stomach seems to be hindered in many HIV+ people early on in infection.

Some factors cited as the cause of these problems include TNF (see pages 198–199) and hydrochloric acid production (see pages 175–176). However, there is little hard evidence of the exact cause of absorption problems, and few documented solutions to this problem. So in this case, as with much of the information on HIV, we are left to keep an eye on our sources of information for future developments in this area.

One point, which is cited repeatedly in the literature, is that HIV+ people, at all stages, need added nutrients (vitamins) to compensate for absorption problems. In addition, they require added sources of protein to supply the raw material for building new cells. In addition to vitamin supplements, I usually recommend a protein shake supplement available in any health-food store.

effects might also hinder the absorption and effectiveness of NAC. If your triglyceride level is high, this probably suggests increased TNF, and possible poor absorption. In these cases, Trental has been shown to lower TNF, and could be taken first, with NAC added after Trental has been started to ensure absorption. Again, when we measure the toxicity of this treatment against its possible benefit, it has "no major adverse reactions," according to the Amsterdam abstract, and that was with intravenous administration, which increases the drug's potency. This evidence supports the use of NAC as a viable option for people putting together a natural-treatment regimen.

As I suggested above, NAC and vitamin C seem to work well together, boosting each other's action and efficacy. The current recommended dose of NAC is

- 1,800 to 2,400 mg a day in 3 or 4 600-mg tablets spread over the day,

though the study abstracted in the Amsterdam report used 3,000 mg intravenously. With the possibility of hindered absorption, higher doses have been discussed. If you plan to pursue higher doses, do so slowly, adding additional pills (one every three days), watching for any adverse effects.

Resources: Estroff Pharmacy by mail order (see Resource Guide); some health-food stores; no prescription necessary.

VITAMIN B$_{12}$

According to a study done by M. K. Baum, et al., for the Sixth International AIDS Conference in San Francisco (abstract F.B.32, reported in *BETA*, November 1990), a significant number of people with HIV infection have a vitamin B$_{12}$ deficiency that results in impaired cognitive function. The report stated that malabsorption of vitamin B$_{12}$ can lead to neurologic disorders. Therefore, the study tested cognitive function. After B$_{12}$ was administered to the patients in the study for six months, test scores of those whose B$_{12}$ status had normalized showed significantly improved scores on tests of cognitive function. The scores of those without this intervention continued to be significantly lower.

Other articles and studies indicate that B$_{12}$ deficiency could be a significant cofactor in HIV nervous system disorders, including peripheral neuropathy. In an article from *Outweek* (June 12, 1991) on B_{12}, Jon M. Greenberg also points out that B_{12} "doesn't appear to have significant toxic side effects, even at doses several times the normal therapeutic dose." Since B_{12} is normally used as treatment for pernicious anemia, under this treatment you might see a rise in your RBC, HGB, and HCT blood values.

An ACT UP treatment alternatives packet contains a handout that cites six different vitamin studies using B_{12}, one in conjunction with AZT, to prevent the possible AZT side effect of anemia. Folate, another nutritional supplement, is also used to treat anemia. If you are anemic, see your doctor. Most physicians use B_{12} and folate together to treat this condition.

Lark Lands, Ph.D., the well-known HIV nutritional researcher, recommends B_{12} as possibly *the* most important supplement for HIV+ people. Also, another B_{12} handout from ACT UP states that peripheral neuropathy can be caused by pernicious anemia and therefore correctible in many cases through treatment with B_{12}.

Vitamin B_{12} is not easily absorbed through the stomach unless it is in a food source. Blue-green algae is a food source of B_{12}, but to attain recommended levels of the vitamin in your system you would need a high-level concentration in the supplement. Intramuscular injections (IM), not oral supplements, are recommended. Some doctors will prescribe needles and a multidose bottle of B_{12} for people to use at home.

Vitamin B_{12} is measured in micrograms (mcg). On a multidose IM injection bottle, the label might say 1,000 mcg/mL, meaning 1,000 micrograms per milliliter. Each mL equals 1 cc on a syringe.

Dosing varies greatly throughout the literature. I recommend B_{12} injections to most clients, even if B_{12} levels are normal. Dosing also varies if the person has anemia or a condition caused by a B_{12} deficiency. Dr. Lands has recommended up to four IM injections per week (IM injections usually measure 1 cc or 1,000 mcg) if a patient is deficient. Then, after the condition has reversed, she recommends continuing with at least two weekly injections. Mainstream medical providers are more conservative and usually give no more than one injection per week. Considering the low toxicity, for people deficient in B_{12}, I agree with Dr. Lands. For those who do not have deficiencies but who wish to include this option in their regimen, one to two IM injections (1 cc per injection) weekly is the recommendation I have experienced positive results with.

If your doctor prescribes self-injection and you have no prior experience with needles, ask the doctor, a nurse, or anyone with experience whom you trust to inject you. To learn how to do it or gain experience, practice—or have your helper practice—on a piece of fruit using water in the syringe. It is a simple task to learn.

Another form of B_{12}, under the brand name Ener-B, is taken intranasally. If you cannot get the shots, this is the next-best choice. It is readily available in any health-food store and comes in packages of ten. Individual dosing tubes contain 400 mcg, which is less than half a shot. The dose should be adjusted to match the recommendations above. But note that Ener-B is probably less efficient, since it is absorbed in the nasal passages. Some practitioners recommend adding a few hundred extra micrograms per dose to compensate for the absorption difference.

Resource: Your local health-food store should have Ener-B. For the injectable, you will need a prescription from your doctor, which is easily filled at your local pharmacy. If you cannot find Ener-B, Estroff Pharmacy, listed in the Resource Guide, has it in stock for mail orders.

HYPERICIN

For about three years, reports have been surfacing as to the benefit of hypericin, a possible antiviral, for HIV infection. Articles in *AIDS Treatment News, BETA, PWA Coalition Newsline,* and *Body Positive* all reported the discovery of hypericin's antiretroviral activity in the test tube. Hypericin is an ingredient in the medicinal herb known as Saint-John's-wort. Eventually, a study on this preparation in HIV patients was done at Community Research Initiative (CRI), and the results were not favorable. Saint-John's-wort didn't harm anyone, but the amount of hypericin it contained did not reach blood concentrations high enough to have any effect against HIV.

A drug company, VimRx, decided to extract hypericin from Saint-John's-wort and create an intravenous preparation to test on humans. The process of extracting the hypericin and subsequently deciding to genetically reproduce it in the lab was time-consuming, to say the least. A new study began in New York (at New York University), Boston, and Minneapolis, in January 1992, approximately three years after the initial discovery of hypericin's activity against HIV. But the research was abruptly discontinued owing to phototoxicity—that is, sensitivity to the sun, varying with the complexion of the participants (light-skinned people were the most sensitive). The first arm of the study was a dose-escalating arm, and the phototoxicity began before the dose was reached that researchers predicted would be effective against HIV. Currently, the study has been started up again, and additional information is not yet available. I would watch for future developments with the IV preparation.

In addition to all these developments with intravenous hypericin, Pacific Biologics, another company, released an oral version of hypericin *extract*. Stronger than Saint-John's-wort, this substance is readily available in pill form at good health-food stores, and phototoxicity does not seem to be a problem. Originally, Pacific Biologics had released a 1.5-mg dose of hypericin extract, which was insufficient for an antiviral effect. Recently, an article in *PWA Newsline* (November 1992, Issue 82) reported on a study published in the journal *Antiviral Research*. The study documented the effectiveness of hypericin against CMV, both in the test tube and in lab animals. This development also suggests antiviral activity against HIV, since it is similar to CMV in that both are lipid-coated viruses. The lipid-coated viruses are the class against which hypericin seems most effective.

In the same *PWA Newsline* article, a report by Forefront Health Investigations recommended 30–100 mg twice a week or 10–20 mg a day as the minimum needed to deactivate viral replication. With Pacific Biologics' recent release of hypericin extract at a dose of 10 mg per capsule, this dosing schedule becomes a more viable option.

• An oral dose of 10 mg taken three times a week would bring you up to the amount where phototoxicity began in the study of intravenous hypericin at New York University, but no phototoxicity has been reported at these doses with the oral preparation.

Hypericin extract is a possible antiviral without severe toxicity. As to dosage, since we now know that 30–100 mg per week, or

10–20 mg per day, seems to be most effective, one should build up slowly, starting with 10 mg three times a week, to watch for phototoxicity. Phototoxicity was not reported with any oral preparation, but building up slowly will offer extra protection. All the while, of course, you must follow your bloodwork.

In *AIDS Treatment News,* hypericin was reported to be possibly useful in combating at least four other viruses. During the CRI study in New York, investigators noticed a positive beneficial effect with respect to hepatitis B. Laboratory tests have also found antiviral activity against CMV, influenza, and human papillomavirus (HPV). One person in the current hypericin trial had an unexpected improvement in genital warts caused by HPV. If you add hypericin to your regimen, keep up on the literature and studies being conducted on this product.

Resource: Oral version available at Estroff Pharmacy by mail order and some health-food stores. You must specify Pacific Biologics' hypericin extract in a 10-mg dose. As I mentioned, the 1.5-mg dose has not shown efficacy.

COMPOSITION A AND ENHANCE (HERBAL MIXTURES)

Composition A is a mixture of twenty-seven Chinese herbs found to have immune-modulating and antiviral capabilities. A small six-month study by David Cohen, an acupuncturist in Los Angeles, used Composition A to treat HIV infection. The results showed significant T4-cell increases in twenty-seven participants who began the study with T4-cell counts above 400. Participants were allowed to take other interventions during the investigation, and no placebo was used as a control. Because of this, mainstream medicine would discount the data collected, citing poor study design.

Nevertheless, since Composition A has a very low toxicity, many have decided to try it for its possible antiviral and immune-modulating capabilities. The amount used in the study was four seven-tablet doses, or seven tablets four times a day. However, some participants developed stomach cramps at this dosage, so the amount was decreased to eliminate the stomach distress. Anecdotal accounts of doses as low as four tablets four times a day are reported as beneficial.

Frank Lipman, M.D., an acupuncturist in New York City, explained his preference over Composition A for another herbal formula, called Enhance. In Chinese medicine, as described in Chapter 7, the practitioner strives to strengthen the kidneys, spleen, and lungs; this, in turn, balances the yin and yang in the body. Enhance has more yin tonics in its formula than Composition A. Dr. Lipman's experience has been that Composition A can often create heat, or a yin deficiency, in patients already yin-deficient. Enhance seems to alleviate yin deficiencies more effectively. Many Chinese-medicine practitioners believe that HIV+ yin deficiencies should not be treated with herbs that create heat.

In addition, the highly regarded Quan Yin Institute in San Francisco, after using Composition A for years with its HIV+ patients, now uses Enhance for the same reasons. In addition, this herbal formula has proven easier to digest than Composition A and contains a greater percentage of blood tonic and vitalizing herbs, which are believed responsible for strengthening the bone marrow that produces an immune-enhancing response.

There is no conclusive research on either product, and both are associated with reports of low toxicity—usually a stomachache, which is rectified by a lowering of the dose. The suggested dose for Enhance is five tablets four times a day. As with Composition A, the study was done with four doses of seven tablets per day, but lower doses have been reported to be effective, and are used when stomach distress is experienced as a side effect.

This intervention seems to have more efficacy for people with T4 cells above 250, but as with any low toxicity option, it can be tried at any point, watching your bloodwork for efficacy.

A new form of Composition A has been released that eliminated heat-causing herbs. The new preparation is simply called Composition. I usually recommend either Enhance or Composition.

Resource: Both are available; and come only in tablet form, from some practitioners (acupuncturists and chiropractors), good health-food stores, and by mail order from Estroff, listed in the Resource Guide. No prescription is needed.

KYOLIC FORMULA 100 OR GARLICIN (GARLIC)

Garlic has long been heralded by natural therapists as a strong antiviral, antifungal, anticandida, antiparasitic, antibacterial, antimicrobial, and anticancer tumor therapy. These effects, though associated with garlic throughout history, have never been scientifically verified, and owing to the inflated cost of the government's scientific verification process, they probably never will be. To verify scientifically the beneficial properties of garlic or any other natural or unnatural substance, someone would have to come along with millions of dollars to set up a trial that the FDA considered scientifically significant. I don't think anyone is coming up with that kind of money to research garlic anytime soon. Instead, we will have to depend on small studies that are scientifically flawed and on our own monitoring methods.

Garlic has been used for centuries as a medicinal herb by many cultures. Nearly since the first HIV cases began appearing, people with HIV have been experimenting with raw cloves of garlic, garlic capsules, and intravenously administered garlic drips. A study in the *Chinese Medicine Journal* suggested intravenous garlic as a treatment for cryptococcal meningitis. The treatment was successful in eleven of the twenty-one cases studied.

Quite recently a client came to me complaining of a parasitic infection. He said he had actually seen small worms swimming in the toilet bowl after a bowel movement. His mother, calling from Puerto Rico, told him he had had such an infection as a child, twenty years ago, and that raw garlic had eliminated the parasites. Before receiving any medical treatment, this patient began a regimen of three to five raw cloves of garlic spread over the day. Within two weeks, there were no visual signs of parasites in his stool. When the doctor realized what had occurred, she insisted on treating the patient for parasites anyway, in case the parasites were hiding up out of the range of where the garlic was being digested. Parasites can lodge in the intestine, where they are difficult to detect and to treat.

Garlic cannot hurt you. Many people complain of the smell, but if you swallow chopped garlic without chewing, as if you were swallowing a pill, no smell of garlic will emanate from your pores and the effect on your breath will be lessened. Alternatively, many pill forms of garlic are available in health-food stores. Two brands, Kyolic Formula 100 and Garlicin, seem to be the most popular and are readily available in pill form at local health-food stores.

Intravenous garlic studies are currently under way, and we should have more information about this treatment soon. This substance certainly shows promise as a treatment for cryptococcal meningitis. And certain specific symptoms would suggest garlic as a possible treatment in HIV people:

• persistent candida or yeast infections
• parasitic infections
• T cells below 100, creating vulnerability to a host of opportunistic infections

A person with these conditions might benefit from using garlic as a prophylaxis or to prevent for fungal infections, but I would not eliminate the mainstream medical interventions while using it.

According to the book *Healing AIDS Naturally* by Laurence Badgley (Human Energy Press, 1987), "a good dose of all garlic is about 0.75 gram/kg of body weight. This works out to about 2.5 ounces of raw garlic cloves for a 180-pound person." Toxicity here is not documented, suggesting no adverse reaction. Recently, an acupuncturist reminded me that garlic produces heat in the body, so people with heat conditions or yin deficiencies should not take garlic. I only recommend its use for parasites and yeast infections.

Resource: Most health-food stores. No prescription required.

FLORA BALANCE OR MEGADOPHILUS (ACIDOPHILUS)

Acidophilus is a naturally occurring intestinal bacterium that is often deficient in people with HIV. The result of this deficiency is yeast infections, both oral and vaginal. Such infections are difficult, though not impossible, to eradicate with acidophilus supplements.

Acidophilus has also been reported to control diarrhea. The best forms of acidophilus seem to be the live ones, often in a liquid. These live substances need to be refrigerated. Two very popular brands of acidophilus are Flora Balance and Mega-dophilus.

If you are currently dealing with a yeast infection, you might want to take an antifungal drug, such as fluconazole (Diflucan) or ketoconazole (Nizoral), to relieve the symptoms of the yeast and then take acidophilus prophylactically, preventing recurrence. Slight yeast infections and even serious ones might be controllable with large doses of acidophilus.

Most people with HIV would benefit from using acidophilus as a prophylaxis, since the substance controls an underlying cofactor, candida. Underlying candida is known to weaken the immune system by consistently engaging it to respond at all stages of HIV infection. In trying to control candida, HIV, and perhaps parasites, the immune system weakens and cannot maintain a sufficient response.

• 2 to 4 capsules before each meal helps to prevent candida problems, but if you currently have candida or diarrhea, you need to take more acidophilus to reestablish the balance in your intestines. For current infection, I recommend mainstream medical treatments followed by high-dose acidophilus prophylaxis.

I recommend acidophilus for everyone across the board. Reducing cofactors leaves the immune system to deal with HIV.

Resource: Your local health-food store. No prescription is needed.

BITTER MELON

Bitter melon is a common herb that is being used by many HIV+s as an antiviral treatment. Its botanical name is *Momordica chrantia,* and its Chinese name is Ku Gua. Bitter melon is a member of the plant family that also includes Compound Q (see Chapter 10). In Chinese medicine, this herb is used for its "cooling influence." Anecdotal reports of efficacy have been published in some AIDS magazines (*PWA Newsline* and *AIDS Treatment News*), but little scientific evidence has been made available on this intervention.

One researcher at New York University isolated a protein,

called MAP-30, from bitter melon. In the test tube, MAP-30 has been found to inhibit HIV replication, inhibit direct cell-to-cell infection, and prevent the formation of the cell clumps known as syncytia (one of the ways HIV seems to destroy cells; see Chapter 2).

Bitter melon has been used orally, but few have seen results from drinking it, at least not before six months of use. The most common way to ingest this herb is through a retention enema (described below), which is easy to self-administer.

For both oral and rectal administration, a tea is prepared from the fruit, leaves, and stems of the bitter melon. It is available fresh between June and October, and can be frozen for out-of-season use. In addition, packages of frozen leaves are imported from the Philippines off-season. At this writing, fresh bitter melon generally costs about a dollar a bunch; frozen leaves are 99 cents to $1.39 per 8-ounce package.

To make a "tea" from bitter melon, simmer three pounds of fruit, leaves, and stems for 25 minutes after bringing the mixture to a boil. You can refrigerate the tea in tight jars for up to ten days.

Drinking the tea exposes it to stomach acid and pancreas enzymes, which can destroy the proteins in the bitter melon; the retention enema is a means of bypassing these substances. This well-established method delivers medication and liquids directly to the colon, the main function of which is to absorb liquid from digestive waste.

The dose for the enema is

- 6 ounces per 100 pounds of body weight,

so a 140-pound person would use 8 ounces per day. If you are using retention enemas for the first time, start with about 4 ounces. First clear the colon with a bowel movement or a warm enema. Then rectally infuse the initial 4 ounces of the tea; you can use an empty Fleet Enema bottle, available at any drugstore. On subsequent days, increase the dose by 2 ounces each day until you achieve the desired dose. After the infusion, you will feel fullness in the colon and an instinctive urge to empty it. If you resist the urge, most of the liquid will be absorbed in one hour.

Some HIV+s use this preparation at night, absorbing the liquid during sleep. Others feel a burst of energy after the treatment, so they cannot administer it at night. Recently, someone using the retention enema advised me that lying in a warm bath caused absorption within ten minutes.

There have been no documented side effects of bitter melon, and the preparation is low in cost. My credo, "Watch your bloodwork," certainly applies here, since T4-cell increases associated with this treatment have been reported.

Treating with bitter melon is not recommended for pregnant women who need syncytia formations.

Resource: This plant is usually available in the neighborhoods or stores that cater to Asians and Pacific Islanders. No prescription is needed.

GLYCERON (GLYCYRRHIZIN)

Glyceron is a tablet manufactured by Minophagen Pharmaceutical Company containing the active ingredient glycyrrhizin. The Japanese have studied glycyrrhizin, an extract from the licorice plant, for its antiviral and immunomodulating activity against HIV and for its effects on liver disease, including hepatitis.

One study reported at the Fifth International Conference on AIDS in Montreal followed twenty asymptomatic HIV+ people. Over the course of two years, of the ten who were given daily oral doses of glycyrrhizin ranging from 150 to 225 mg, none progressed to symptoms. In the control group of ten, three progressed to AIDS, two of whom died.

And in one anecdotal self-report, an HIV+ man claims that his T4 cells went from below 50 to 800 on an intravenous preparation of glycyrrhizin. Such dramatic results have not been duplicated with the oral preparation, but the company claims that long-term oral use would yield the same benefits.

Glycyrrhizin is relatively nontoxic, but it does have some side effects. These include hypokalemia (low potassium levels), myopathy (muscle soreness or fatigue), high blood pressure, and sodium and fluid retention. People with high blood pressure are not advised to use this option. Also, those who do use this treatment must have potassium blood levels taken every two weeks for the first two months. If potassium levels drop, discontinue use.

For adults, the suggested dose is

• 2 to 3 tablets a day taken orally after meals. There is an intravenous preparation, but currently it is not widely available.

Resource: The DAAIR buyers club (see Resource Guide) in New York has this product in stock. Also check with the other buyers clubs listed in the Resource Guide.

A prescription is necessary for distribution.

BETA-CAROTENE AND VITAMIN A

Beta-carotene makes vitamin A in the body. But unlike vitamin A, beta-carotene can be taken in high doses without toxicity. According to the book *Healing AIDS Naturally,* "beta-carotene has been shown to protect the immune system of animals treated with immune-suppressive drugs and steroids."

Many natural practitioners and all the natural-medicine literature talk about the benefits of beta-carotene as an antiviral and anticancer supplement. Lark Lands, in her report "The Therapeutic Basics for People Living with HIV," recommends 10,000 to 25,000 IU (international units) of vitamin A daily. Because of digestive problems experienced by some HIV+ individuals, she suggests a water-soluble form. She also states, "Sufficient levels of vitamin A are critical for disease resistance and immune function."

Beta-carotene seems to be a nontoxic form of vitamin A and a preferable choice for this therapy. Lands suggests both, with beta-carotene or carotene complex (a superior drug form; brands are not specified here) at doses of from 10,000 to 50,000 IU per day. Blue-green algae is high in beta-carotene, and often a supplement is unnecessary.

Remember, vitamin A is toxic. Before using supplements of this vitamin, do some research or check with a professional who has knowledge of vitamin supplements.

Resource: Both vitamin A and beta-carotene are available in many brands at good health-food stores, and salespeople can help you select from among the brands. No prescription is necessary.

VITAMIN E

Among the most common skin problems in HIV infection are psoriasis and seborrhea. When taken internally, vitamin E seems to have some positive effect on these conditions by moisturizing the skin. In addition, many naturalists believe that vitamin E is a "free-radical scavenger," meaning that it reduces free radicals in the blood. The theory is that free radicals create an environment in which viruses can grow more readily.

The recommended dose is

• 400 to 800 units daily.

According to Dr. Michelle Alpert, larger doses are not recommended and are linked to viral exacerbation rather than reduction.

Resource: Any health-food store. No prescription is needed. Water-soluble pills are the form most often recommended.

THIOCTIC ACID

Two reports—one in the health-care section of an issue of *NYQ* (January 6, 1992) and one created by Vic Hernandez from ten studies chronicling the possible benefits of thioctic acid—claim that thioctic acid protects the liver from toxic medication by helping it produce more enzymes to manage the toxins.

If your SGOT and SGPT levels are elevated, this liver-protection agent might help lower those enzymes. In addition, it may protect you from toxic effects of medication. The recommended dose is

• a 100-mg capsule three times a day, with meals.

Resource: Available at good health-food stores or Estroff Pharmacy. No prescription is needed.

PHYLLMARTIN (HERBAL PREPARATION)

Phyllmartin is a new herbal preparation by Planter Amica for which there is very little research. What literature exists on this substance claims activity with hepatitis B and C and the HIV virus. I have used phyllmartin with no reports of toxicity in three patients with chronic hepatitis and liver enzymes elevated way above normal—SGOT and SGPT at 500 to 800. In all of these cases, the liver enzymes were down to normal within two months.

Chronic hepatitis seems to be common with HIV infection, and is a serious problem that can result in a shortened life for HIV+ people. This consideration—plus the fact that the mainstream treatment for chronic hepatitis, alpha interferon, can have serious side effects—makes phyllmartin a significant option.

The recommended dose is

• one pill three times a day for two months.

Resource: Estroff Pharmacy or a good herbal pharmacy. No prescription required.

L-LYSINE

Two Indiana University researchers, Dr. Arthur Norins and Dr. Richard Griffith, have reported that taking extra amounts of the amino acid L-lysine suppresses the herpes virus. Results obtained from some 250 herpes patients show that this treatment prevents recurrent lesions. Two other studies, "Subjective Response to Lysine in the Therapy of Herpes Simplex" (45 subjects—published in the *Journal of Antimicrobial Chemotherapy*, 1983, issue 12) and "A Multicentered Study of Lysine Therapy in Herpes Simplex Infection" (1,543 subjects—published in *Dermatologics*, 1978, issue 156), concluded that lysine prevented recurrence, decreased the frequency of infection, and speeded up recovery from a herpes infection.

Since herpes is a cofactor in the progression of HIV infection, I usually recommend L-lysine as a prophylaxis treatment with people who have any history of herpes, including chickenpox, and who have approximately 350 or more T cells.

The dose of L-lysine is

- 1,500 mg daily, usually in three 500-mg-tablet doses.

Some practitioners recommend up to 6 grams of lysine, which is 6,000 mg. When doses exceed 3 grams (3,000 mg), cholesterol levels should be monitored, since lysine may stimulate the liver to increase its manufacture of this substance. No other toxicities were found.

Resource: Available at most health-food stores. No prescription needed.

SHARK CARTILADE (SHARK CARTILAGE)

For years shark cartilage has been studied as a cancer treatment with some positive results. Most recently two articles stimulated new interest in this treatment specifically for people with KS. Michael Callen, a long-term survivor of AIDS, chronicled his experience in one article in *NYQ* claiming a total KS remission when he combined shark cartilage with his radiation treatments.

In addition, angiogenesis, the process by which the body makes new blood vessels, is hindered by shark cartilage. KS needs new blood vessels to grow, and angiogenesis inhibitors, now in drug trials, have been touted as "the cure" for KS. Unfortunately, early trials show high toxicity for the chemical angiogenesis inhibitors.

Shark cartilage does not seem to have much toxicity. In addition, this has long been a "natural" remedy for arthritis. My mother used the cartilage and has almost completely recovered from crippling arthritis.

Resource: Available in any good health-food store or Estroff Pharmacy without a prescription. The shark cartilage needs to be taken for long periods (one to two years, according to some reports) to be effective in controlling KS. The manufacturer recommends starting with approximately 20 pills per day for the first two weeks, and then using 6 to 10 pills daily, indefinitely.

GOZARTE AND UDARTE (KNOWN ONLY BY THESE BRAND NAMES)

These two herbs are used by physicians and natural treatment practitioners to combat parasitic infections and, occasionally, candidiasis (thrush). I have dealt with many HIV patients who suffered from diarrhea and who were later diagnosed with parasites. Testing for parasites consists of a stool sample, usually taken after the patient ingests some type of laxative. These stool tests are often inaccurate, however, and can read negative even when a patient is infected. Some doctors say these stool tests have a 50 percent false-negative rate.

These herbs are usually free of side effects. In the manufacturer's literature no side effects are cited, but there is a recommendation not to use during pregnancy or by couples who intend to conceive. The reason for this recommendation is not given.

Gozarte and Udarte can often minimize the side effects of parasite-fighting drugs. Parasitic infections thrive in some HIV+ people, causing undue stress on the immune system. The drug flagyl is used to treat parasites such as amoebiases, E. coli, and hominis. Besides being ineffective much of the time, flagyl also has side effects that can include nausea and dizziness. In addition, while flagyl eliminates the parasite, it also eliminates beneficial flora needed to control thrush, resulting in thrush or yeast infections. Since Udarte and Gozarte are effective in fighting thrush, this side effect is eliminated. These herbs are usually combined to assure elimination of the infection.

Resource: There is no prescription necessary and they are both available through Estroff Pharmacy. The usual dose is 3 capsules of each per day (6 capsules total), alternating Gozarte with Udarte, 1 every three hours. That is, take Gozarte first, then Udarte three hours later, and repeat until 3 Gozarte and 3 Udarte capsules have been consumed. It does not matter which herb you take first, as long as you alternate them. Usual treatment time is six weeks. The therapy is usually continued in a reduced dosage (2 of each per day) one month after symptom resolution or a stool sample reads negative.

OXYGEN THERAPY

This is a therapy that I have little experience with, but I felt it was important to include it since there have been anecdotal reports of its effectiveness.

The book listed in the Resource Guide, *Oxygen Therapies,* by Ed McCabe (Energy Publications), contains extensive information on oxygen therapy, though most of the information is based on experience with cancer. The therapy itself consists of drinking small amounts of food-grade hydrogen peroxide. As I said, my experience with this is limited, so please consult the book before talking to your physician if you are interested in this treatment. This is a less toxic treatment, without many reports of side effects. No prescription is needed.

OZONE THERAPY

Upon completion of the final updates for this book in February 1993, there were a few reports of benefit from ozone therapy; as a result, a large number of HIV+ people have taken an interest in this treatment. Since many of my own consultation clients began requesting information on this therapy, I began to research its efficacy.

In August of 1992, I requested and received a report from Medizone International Inc., the drug company which was seeking FDA approval for human trials of ozone therapy. This therapy, according to Steven Hillyer, who has produced a documentary on the subject, simply consists of removing blood from an HIV+ person, adding ozone gas to the removed blood to kill off the HIV virus, and then reinfusing the "healthy" blood back into the donor. The Medizone report included research by Dr. Bernard Poiesz that stated ozone treatment resulted in "100 percent inactivation of the virus" while maintaining the health of other blood cells.

According to Steven Hillyer, there are three ways this therapy is being used:

- 500 ccs of blood are removed from the HIV+ person, ozone gas is injected and mixed into the bagged blood, the blood is reinfused.

- 20 ccs of blood are removed from the HIV+ person into a syringe, where the ozone gas is added, mixed, and the blood is reinfused.
- An ozone generator is purchased for approximately $2,200, and the gas is administered rectally, several times per week.

Mr. Hillyer pointed out to me that nutritional supplements, vitamin-C drips, and dietary modifications were necessary for the best results. I suggested to Mr. Hillyer that these alterations alone, quite possibly, could stall HIV progression.

Although this procedure is being "talked up" in the underground treatment circles, there are no studies that confirm the few anecdotal reports of efficacy that exist. In addition, this procedure has been used for years in Germany and other European countries as an AIDS treatment. Personally, I heard about this treatment five years ago, and subsequently heard that benefit was transient and nonconfirmed. If a treatment was being used for over five years and people were being treated with great effectiveness, I believe more reports of efficacy would be generated. I personally suggest waiting for more information on this one.

There are many alternative practitioners who are using ozone therapy, and calling your local HIV community-based organization should help get a resource if you wish to explore this treatment.

SUMMARY

No matter which intervention you use, you need to monitor your blood results. Don't make a plan that includes everything in this chapter. If you do, you won't be able to tell what's working. Instead, make a plan that contains two antivirals, two immune modulators, and nutrients taken as needed. Since most of these options are nontoxic and can usually be mixed without worry, check with a practitioner and then try different combinations.

It is hard to be precise, since HIV is not an exact science. At the health facility for HIV+ people where I used to work, the pharmacist is constantly questioning the doctor on her varying combinations of therapies, attempting to pin her down on a "standard" practice. *But we do not have enough information on HIV infection to identify a standard practice*. However, one thing *is* certain: the more natural options take longer to work (six months to a year).

Some natural interventions that have been touted as HIV treatments but are not covered here include aloe vera juice, Iscador, coenzyme Q-10, lentinen, and KM. You'll need to research these options on your own. I have not found enough supportive information on them to suggest that they are effective. Project Inform's hot line, listed in the Resource Guide, is the perfect first telephone call for anyone seeking information about treatment options.

Finding a support group in which you can share information and follow other people on different treatments is always beneficial—not only to support and boost faith in your treatments but also to enrich your overall life. But you can help yourself to believe in your treatment choices as well by using affirmations like these:

- "I believe in my treatments."
- "All the treatments I take work on me perfectly."
- "All the treatments I choose are perfect treatments for controlling HIV in my body."
- "These treatments heal my body and support my immune system."
- "My T4 cells are constantly increasing."
- "I welcome perfect health."

Believe in the treatments you choose.

Immune Modulators

All doctors involved in the treatment of HIV infection appear to agree in theory that HIV treatment must be approached in two ways:

- with an antiviral, to stop the virus;
- and with an immune modulator, to increase the action of the immune system and in some cases help rebuild it, as evidenced by a T4-cell count rise.

As a matter of fact, conferences have been held specifically on immune modulation and rebuilding the immune system. As yet, no drugs have been endorsed by the FDA specifically for immune modulation. But certain drugs, already approved by the FDA for other purposes, have been shown to be effective in modulating the immune system and increasing the T4-cell count. In my opinion, these drugs, which are low in toxicity, are not used often enough, even when they appear to be related to increases in T4-cell counts.

IMMUTHIOL (DTC)

In an early French study of Immuthiol, the brand name of the drug DTC, which involved six people in 1985, all but one showed clinical improvements—including T4-cell increases and an increased sensitivity in skin tests (anergy panel) that measure the strength of the immune-system response. After the drug was discontinued, the improvements disappeared. Also, in 1987 a study of twenty-six patients at the University of Arizona showed that Immuthiol slowed the progression of HIV-related symptoms. At the conclusion of the study, the investigators recommended that AZT be combined with Immuthiol.

A French placebo-controlled study of ninety HIV-symptomatic patients yielded impressive clinical laboratory improvements with no significant side effects. Specifically, subjects showed an average T-cell increase of 169. However, researchers believed that as much as a 30-percent change in T-cell count, either up or down, could be attributed to other fluctuating factors, so in this study the T-cell increases were not judged clinically significant.

In 1988, doctors in New York began giving patients Antabuse (a drug used to treat alcoholism), which, according to earlier research, in the body turns into DTC, the main ingredient in Immuthiol. Anecdotal reports of the efficacy of Antabuse ranged from incredible to nonexistent. Some doctors gave this treatment across the board. Others dismissed it as a hoax. And a few progressive physicians advised patients that since the toxicity of Antabuse was minimal, and since it worked on some but not all people, the drug was certainly worth a try.

In October 1990, New Zealand licensed Immuthiol (DTC) as a treatment for HIV-infected people in whom AZT therapy was ineffective. Buyers clubs throughout the nation started to ship this drug into the United States for individual purchase. In March of that year, Merieux, the French drug company that owned the patent on Immuthiol, had submitted a treatment IND application—an application for an "investigational new drug"— to the FDA. Approval of the application would have allowed Merieux to test this drug in humans, but the FDA turned Merieux down, citing insufficient evidence of efficacy in the laboratory. A few months after the FDA's denial and New Zealand's acceptance of the drug, a report released by Merieux, later included in the abstracts for the 1992 Eighth International AIDS Conference in Amsterdam, cited Immuthiol as nonbeneficial and announced that the company was taking the drug off the market.

With all the evidence of Immuthiol's positive effects, the company's announcement that the drug was ineffective took the AIDS-treatment world aback. My response was to begin my own personal investigation. I spoke with a doctor who had acted as a consultant to the Merieux board of directors. I was told that Merieux had decided to cut its losses and remove the drug from the shelves, after an inside source had reported that the FDA would never approve Immuthiol in the United States. There has been no corroboration of this.

If true, this story would be a classic example of how the FDA's regulatory process may be politically motivated and may interfere with the search for effective treatments and cures, since it was suggested to me that the FDA's reasoning was that availability of AZT in the country made it unnecessary to provide access to Immuthiol. But AZT is approved as an antiviral, and Immuthiol appears to work as an immune modulator. Even though these decisions are confusing and disappointing, we must not stop exploring *all* our options, whether they are sanctioned by the government or not. Our lives are at stake, and any treatment that can possibly offer benefit should be available for exploration!

ANTABUSE (DISULFIRAM)

With just about no toxicity, Antabuse—a drug developed to treat alcoholism by causing an allergic reaction to alcohol—is an immune-modulating option. According to the manufacturer, for reasons not fully understood roughly 64 percent of Antabuse is converted into DTC in the bloodstream. Others put the figure at 90 percent. In any case, Antabuse has been used by many patients. In addition, CRI (Community Research Initiative), which does small community-based drug trials, has monitored and collected data from people on the drug. On a dose of 500 mg twice weekly in tablet form, many patients had a significant—greater than 30 percent—increase in T_4 cells. The earlier the stage of HIV infection, the greater the benefit seems to be. Those people with AIDS who took Antabuse had less significant T_4-cell increases. However, considering the low toxicity of the drug, Antabuse is worth trying at any stage of infection.

Bernard Bihari, M.D., a leading HIV doctor and researcher, claims that even if T_4-cell counts do not rise, many people who take Antabuse, naltrexone, and Tagamet, three of the more popular immune modulators, develop fewer opportunistic infections than those who do not.

Promising Treatments and the FDA

The FDA's process of drug approval is stringent, political, conservative—even in cases of death by illness—and expensive. Some drug companies spend up to one billion dollars to test and ultimately market products in the United States. This well-known fact supports the argument that a company has a financial incentive to pull even a promising drug from the market when it starts becoming clear that it will fail to win government approval.

One of the intriguing aspects of the 1992 AIDS conference in Amsterdam was the fact that each exhibition booth on the conference floor had testing procedures and new drugs planned for release in many countries prior to their ultimate release in the United States. I believe, as many others do, that the FDA needs to reassess its drug-approval process and redefine its procedures, especially in potentially life-threatening situations.

My immediate concern is that the FDA is looking to seize natural substances and to limit the right of vitamin makers and herb suppliers to sell their products and claim them beneficial. If the FDA decides that it should test and label all the products that go on the market, it will put hundreds of small manufacturers out of business and therefore throw the economy into an even greater tailspin than we are currently experiencing. If the FDA decides to enter the vitamin industry, the big drug companies will get larger, the doctors will get richer, and people seeking alternative therapy benefits will suffer tremendously. The market will be limited and most of the drugs now readily available will go underground, which means quality will suffer and prices will rise.

This is an important time for contacting your legislators. Tell them how you feel about the ultimate FDA approval and status of vitamins and natural medicinal interventions.

As concerned as I am about this issue, it's important not to minimize the progress within the FDA under the leadership of David Kessler, M.D. Dr. Kessler inherited a problematic approval process and made significant efforts to update and streamline the agency's policies. His admirable efforts have benefited the HIV community notably, and I urge him to continue his progressive management of the FDA. I also urge *you* to make your feelings known to Dr. Kessler. Write to him and encourage him to continue to relax the policies that block promising treatments from reaching those who need them.

With just about no toxicity, Antabuse is an immune-modulating option. The side effects include:

- a metallic taste
- an allergic reaction to alcohol consumption (and, for some, mouthwash or cologne; you need to test your own sensitivity)
- stomach cramps, which are easily avoided by taking the drug on a full stomach

The dose that has been shown to be beneficial is

- a 500-mg tablet twice a week.

Twenty-four to forty-eight hours after ingestion of Antabuse, most people can ingest alcohol without any reaction. One woman I knew took Antabuse for three years, stabilizing her T4-cell count at between 400 and 500. Her employment required that she work with photography chemicals, and her hands were often in alcohol, but she experienced no reaction whatsoever. So each person responds individually—just as HIV manifests itself differently in every person.

Antabuse, with its low toxicity and possible benefit to T4-cell increases, is an early intervention to try if T4 cells are consistently decreasing. This option can be used with AZT or before AZT, which is much more toxic. It is recommended for people with T4 cells between 100 and 600; a prescription from your doctor is required.

TREXAN (NALTREXONE HYDROCHLORIDE)

Naltrexone hydrochloride is the drug, not the product, name; most of the literature refers to this treatment as naltrexone, so I do the same here. Most of the research to date done on naltrexone has been conducted by a single researcher, Dr. Bernard Bihari, and his colleagues. He has presented his findings at international AIDS conferences, but has not as yet published them in a major medical journal. Dr. Bihari's evidence stems from the theory that hormones regulate immune function and endorphin (a hormone that regulates pain) is a principal part of

Testing Your Antabuse Sensitivity

Some people are so extremely sensitive to Antabuse that after taking it they respond adversely to a topical product containing alcohol. Some people, though, have no reaction. If you take Antabuse and wish to use cologne or mouthwash, then a few hours after taking Antabuse, place a tiny little drop of either of these two substances on your skin:

• If it burns, do not use the product. You are extremely sensitive.

• If no burning occurs, try a larger drop on the skin. If still no burning occurs, your sensitivity to Antabuse is minimal and you can use cologne. Mouthwash is still not recommended until thirty-six hours after the Antabuse dose. After that, slowly test oral sensitivity in the same manner, starting with a single drop.

Consuming alcohol under any circumstances is definitely not recommended.

that regulation. When a person ingests naltrexone before bedtime, endorphin production, which occurs during sleep, is increased, which in turn increases the function of immune cells and possibly increases T4-cell counts.

Naltrexone was a drug developed as a treatment to block the effects of opiate drugs, such as heroin. Doses of 50 mg to 100 mg are used for substance abusers, but for immune-modulating purposes only a very small amount of naltrexone,

• 3 mg daily at bedtime (the preparation is usually a cough medicine–like syrup made from 50 mg pills)

is used to stimulate endorphin production. There are side effects related to naltrexone use—for example, elevated liver enzymes—but they do not seem to manifest at a dose of only 3 mg daily.

Again, because of its low toxicity and possible benefit, it is a viable option, well worth a try. In my clinical experience, I have seen both Antabuse and naltrexone work to stimulate T4-cell production, and as I wrote earlier, both seem to work best when

T4 cells are above 200. But both are worth a try no matter where you are along the spectrum of HIV infection, as long as you are monitoring your bloodwork.

You must be careful with the preparation of naltrexone, since a liquid low-dose (3 mg nightly) preparation is not available from the manufacturer and must be mixed by a pharmacist. Many pharmacies across the country have been mixing naltrexone regularly for their patients and make good, balanced mixtures. The Resource Guide lists a pharmacy that accepts phone orders with credit cards and has a history of mixing naltrexone for this purpose. You can ask a pharmacist if he has experience mixing this 3 mg preparation. A prescription is required for naltrexone.

TAGAMET (CIMETIDINE)

This drug, approved by the FDA for treating peptic ulcers, has shown more clinical evidence than naltrexone and Antabuse of immune-modulating capabilities. According to a German trial by N. Brockmeyer, M.D., and colleagues, increases in T4 levels do not occur at 800 mg a day of Tagamet but are seen clearly at 1,600 mg a day. Dr. Bihari reports that on Tagamet, one patient's T4-cell count went from 156 to 511 in three months and then to 684 in six months. When the drug was discontinued, the T4-cell count began to revert.

Experience with Tagamet among my clients has been extremely positive. One client on the drug went from 400 T4 cells to 1,200 in one year. Since the drug is also used for peptic ulcers, long-term use does not seem to be extremely toxic, but you must discuss toxicity with your doctor prior to taking *any* medication and be closely monitored for toxicity once you have begun to take the medication. Side effects can include diarrhea, nausea, vomiting, muscle pain, and, in a small percentage of people, decreased libido and possible impotence.

Frank Lipman, M.D., has pointed out that some practitioners believe Tagamet may cause absorption problems, which already exist in many HIV+s. Tagamet decreases the hydrochloric acid production in the stomach, one of the digestive acids; some practitioners believe absorption problems are often caused by lack of hydrochloric acid. Therefore, Tagamet could exacerbate absorption problems. This should certainly be a consideration in making a decision regarding the option. Some practitioners suggest a hydrochloric acid supplement, available at health-food stores, to be taken with each meal while on this therapy. This might alleviate any absorption problems Tagamet might cause.

Since Tagamet affects the pH balance in the stomach, it might also interfere with the digestion of certain drugs, such as dapsone, which is used to prevent PCP. Therefore, Dr. Bihari recommends that, during Tagamet treatment, dapsone dose be increased by 50 percent.

For immune modulation, the recommended dose for Tagamet, which is a prescription drug available in tablet form, is

- 400 mg four times a day, to equal 1,600 mg daily.

The preceding three immune modulators discussed—Antabuse, naltrexone, and Tagamet—have been widely discussed in the HIV literature. Most doctors in New York City, San Francisco, and Los Angeles are aware of the possible benefits of these drugs and readily prescribe them *at a patient's request.* If your doctor is not aware of the information on these three immune modulators, you can contact Project Inform for packets of information for each of them. Simply dial the 800 number for Project Inform (see the Resource Guide) and request that the packets be mailed to you. If your doctor is unaware of this information, it might be time for him or her to do some reading.

GAMMAR-IV OR GAMULIN (HUMAN IMMUNE GLOBULIN)

In most listings, this treatment is referred to as gamma globulin. This term is a combination of a brand and drug name: the brand name for the intravenous preparation is Gammar-IV, and that for the intramuscular preparation is Gamulin, while the actual drug contained in these products is human immune globulin.

A 1986 issue of *AIDS Treatment News* contained a report on a study from the Albert Einstein College of Medicine that outlined the benefits of gamma-globulin treatment. And in 1988, a study was completed by J. B. Bussel, M.D., and his colleagues on the benefits of gamma globulin in HIV patients with ITP (idiopathic thrombocytopenic purpura), or low blood platelets. These two reports, and the content of gamma globulin itself, led many doctors to try different amounts and different preparations of gamma globulin—either intravenous (IV) or intramuscular injection (IM)—as a means of boosting their HIV+ patients' immune systems.

Gamma globulin is a blood product that is extremely rich in antibodies, the backbone of the immune system. This antibody-rich substance has been around for quite a while and has been used to treat viral hepatitis, measles, rubella, and hypogammaglobulinemia. In a pediatric study, 42 percent of the treatment group had T-cell count improvement, compared to 7 percent of the control group. Anecdotal reports seemed to confirm that T-cell increases in adults were also a possible result of gamma-globulin treatment.

This promising information resulted in great demand for gamma globulin among HIV+ adults. The run on the product began in 1991 and peaked at the start of 1992, when the supplier announced a possible shortage of gamma globulin. Dr. Michelle Alpert, one of the doctors who subscribed to gamma globulin treatment and who had administered more than 200 gamma-globulin infusions, reported possible benefits from the infusions early on. However, after several months of treating patients with gamma globulin, benefit was inconsistent—in some patients T4 cells rose and in others counts remained unchanged. The reports published for the 1992 Amsterdam conference were also mixed.

According to one abstract from the Amsterdam conference report (PoB 3452), gamma-globulin treatment yielded "some clinical benefit in adult patients with AIDS," while another (PoB 3454) said "data does not support IVIG [another way gamma globulin is identified] use with advanced disease." These studies gave further evidence to the trend that Dr. Alpert and I both noted among our clients—the treatment was effective in some cases but not all. And since the second abstract did not show benefit with IV gamma-globulin use in advanced disease, the possibility that the treatment is more beneficial early on becomes a real and worthy possibility for further investigation.

It makes sense that gamma globulin, which is rich in antibodies, would help support a stifled immune system in fighting everyday infections and possibly keeping people symptom-free for longer periods of time. In addition, several patients whom I have personally chronicled have benefited from gamma globulin with significant T4-cell rises. One woman's T4 cells went from 250 to 550 over a six-month period of consistent (weekly) IVIG treatments. Unfortunately, the T4 cells began to decrease when weekly infusions were discontinued.

Since gamma globulin is extremely expensive, insurance companies by and large pressure medical scientists *not* to test this product further on adults. Widespread use would so tax the system that the insurance industry would suffer greatly. This is another sad weakness of our current health-care system— avoiding possible beneficial treatments because of their expense. How can we put a price on human life?

According to a report in *AIDS Treatment News*, one doctor gave a 2-cc intramuscular injection of gamma globulin weekly to patients with fewer than 500 T-helper cells. This is a less expensive way of giving gamma globulin than the IV preparation, and the doctor reported fewer opportunistic infections and possible stabilization of T4 cells.

Because gamma globulin is a blood product, it has no toxicities at all, but some people are allergic to the intravenous preparation and have to be given epinephrine or Benadryl during the IV drip. Therefore, the first infusion of this product must be closely monitored. Since this allergic reaction can result in anaphylactic shock (a drop in blood pressure and breathing impairment), many doctors overreact, claiming severe problems with this possible side effect. But since allergic reactions are both very rare and easily reversed when they occur if the patient is monitored, and since there are no toxicities to organs or blood associated with this product, gamma globulin remains an efficient and highly beneficial immune-modulating possibility.

In addition, IV gamma globulin has been demonstrated to be effective in the treatment of HIV-related ITP (low platelets). When a person's platelet count is deteriorating, this treatment is called for early on (when the platelet count drops below 70,000) to avoid the use of other, toxic drugs, such as prednisone, later in the progression of ITP.

A 2-cc intramuscular injection of gamma globulin is inexpensive and has no side effects. I recommend this intervention at any point in the progression of HIV infection. Patients report feeling energized and that rashes, swollen glands, fevers, and diarrhea sometimes resolve. Another product, called hyperimmune globulin, contains HIV antibodies and might be more effective for people who are HIV+; but it is not yet available. Trials on this nontoxic preparation are promising.

People who take IV gamma globulin should consult their doctors about dosage as related to their body weight. Most people take carefully monitored infusions of

- either 12 grams (two 6-gram bottles),
- or, for people over 200 pounds, 18 grams (three 6-gram bottles).

The recommendations in the *Physicians' Desk Reference,* the standard resource for prescription drugs, are to infuse patients with a loading dose, which consists of weekly infusions of gamma globulin, and then observe a 28-day waiting period between treatments. The system appears to be depleted of antibodies, which the gamma globulin is rich in, after the 28-day period.

Most doctors try to work through insurance companies in providing this treatment. For the IV preparation, a prescription is usually provided to the patient, who then secures the gamma globulin at the local pharmacy and returns to the doctor's office to have it administered. Doctors usually have the IM (immune-modulating) shots available in their offices.

NEUPOGEN (FILGRASTIM)

This new injectable drug can dramatically increase white blood cell counts. My professional experience with Neupogen has been extraordinary. One patient on Neupogen with a WBC count of 1.0 had an increase to 7.0 within two weeks; two others had similar increases.

Neupogen is administered by injection and a prescription is needed. The one drawback to this useful treatment is its exorbitant price. If your white blood cell count is low, a condition commonly called neutropenia, this is probably the best available treatment.

SUMMARY

Immune-modulating therapies are currently limited—we need aggressive exploration and research in this area. Certainly, AIDS activists and doctors alike have been calling for more such research, but their cries have been totally disregarded, even though experts agree that immune modulation will be very important in restoring people's immune systems. Political action groups, such as ACT UP, are pivotal in pressuring researchers in a certain direction and are a good venue for people frustrated by the system.

In the preceding section, I referred to hyperimmunotherapy, also called passive immune therapy. In this treatment, healthy HIV+ donors give their blood, which is separated and processed to kill any infectious agents, frozen, and mixed with other HIV+ antibody solutions. This process gives the substance a wide range of antibodies from several different donors. The preparation is then infused into people with AIDS.

Passive immune therapy has been studied off and on for the last five years. Unfortunately, the studies have focused only on people seriously ill with extremely progressed HIV infection. I always wonder whether the effects of the intervention would have been more beneficial if they had been administered sooner. In any case, passive immunotherapy is difficult to get and is mostly confined to studies. One doctor, listed in the Resource Guide, separates the blood and infuses people himself. If you are interested in this therapy, read the resources and call the doctor for further information.

Other potential immune modulators are DHEA, tacrine, thymotrinin, MEK (methionine enkephalin), trentalpentox, and NAC (these are all drug or substance names; brand and company names are not yet available). Small studies have suggested that each of these drugs has some small immune-modulating properties.

In summary, I can only urge you to do your research:

- Call your local community-based organization for any information on the substance you are considering.
- Call Project Inform for an information packet.

- Call GMHC's *Treatment Issues* or John James's *AIDS Treatment News* for specific issues devoted to the treatment you're interested in.

Then begin your treatment routine methodically by taking these steps:

- Get a baseline bloodwork—a bloodwork taken before you begin this regimen.
- Monitor your bloodwork as outlined in Chapter 5.

This book will not cover every available intervention. It is impossible to do that, since the information changes every day. But it does refer you to all the resources you need to keep yourself updated with the latest treatment information. By reading the articles you track down, you'll be able to make informed treatment decisions. Include your doctor in the process—and this I recommend highly. Get your doctor's input, keep the doctor updated on the information you're collecting, and by all means get the doctor to participate fully in monitoring the treatment's efficacy.

There is one more benefit to keeping yourself informed—one that is less evident than the others. Fear often helps us make decisions that are radical and even dangerous, and that same fear can sometimes interfere with the decision-making process. Perhaps the most powerful means you have of diminishing that fear is the gathering of information. The more information you gather, the more empowered and in control you will feel. Of course, there is *always* some uncertainty about whether a treatment option will work. The challenge is to keep a positive thought—"The treatment is working"—in the same mental space holding the resolve that if it doesn't you will methodically go on to other options.

For many people, death lies at the root of fear. And the fact is that you are facing a challenging, possibly life-threatening disease. But the only reason you are so concerned with death as an HIV+ person is that you have learned that you have a virus. In the past, the possibility that you could die tomorrow, even without the virus, existed as well. People die in car accidents, in plane accidents, of cancer, and of heart attacks every day of the week, but they are in denial of the fact that death is a possibility for them every day. HIV pushes people out of that denial—and that accounts for the fear.

Remember, everyone on the planet is facing the possibility of death tomorrow. Put it in perspective. Don't let the possibility become an overwhelming mountain; it can be just another reality that you factor in with the rest.

One of my favorite aphorisms comes from Alcoholics Anonymous: "Fear is lack of faith." That says it all.

CHAPTER 10

Antiviral Options

The antiviral option (or options) within your treatment regimen should inhibit the progression of HIV infection. An antiviral is a drug or natural substance that is effective in either stopping the growth of or eliminating a virus—in this case, the HIV virus. Since HIV is a retrovirus, the antivirals used to treat HIV infection are called antiretrovirals. As I explained in Chapter 2, retroviruses replicate in a manner that is actually the opposite of what we consider normal. Ordinarily, the reproductive function begins with DNA, which requires RNA to replicate. However, the HIV virus begins with RNA, and converts DNA to RNA to replicate. This classifies HIV as a retrovirus, and HIV is the first retrovirus found in humans. Prior to this discovery, retroviruses had been found in animals only.

Again, to reiterate briefly (for a complete review, reread Chapter 2): When HIV is replicating, it uses a series of genes and enzymes to complete the process. One of the major enzymes involved in this replication process is reverse transcriptase. This enzyme converts DNA into RNA, allowing the virus to use the RNA for replication purposes. All of the antiretrovirals currently approved by the FDA for treating HIV infection—AZT, ddI, and ddC—inhibit reverse transcription, or, in other words, block reverse transcriptase. These three drugs are categorized as *nucleoside analogues,* and are available by prescription only.

Other genes involved in the replication process are TAT and

GAG. TAT gene inhibitors are currently being researched and look promising as antiretrovirals for HIV infection. As you must know by now, I believe we are on the brink of discovering treatments that will give HIV-infected people normal life expectancy. But in the meantime, we must bridge the gap by using what treatments we have.

I discuss the nucleoside analogues in this chapter first, since they are so widely used—and, in my opinion, both misused and abused as well. Remember, an antiviral is an important part of your regimen, but there are natural antivirals, produced from such substances as herbs, that have little or no toxicity. (For information on these natural interventions, see Chapter 8.) You may want to try these before turning to these more aggressive, more toxic treatments, especially if you are currently asymptomatic with T4 cells above 350 or 400.

RETROVIR OR AZT (ZIDOVUDINE)

A word on the terminology: Retrovir is the brand name of the drug zidovudine. This product has come to be known as AZT.

If you are struggling with the decision to start AZT, it's important for you to research the drug and its potential side effects. The *AmFAR Directory,* Project Inform, GMHC's *Treatment Issues,* and John James's *AIDS Treatment News*—all listed in Chapter 19, Keeping Current, under Periodicals—provide overviews on AZT studies and their results. This drug has received a lot of negative press, mostly due to long-term toxicity and side effects. The toxicity of AZT includes lowered red and white blood counts, and side effects are nausea, fatigue and/or depression, abdominal pain, and severe headaches. These side effects often resolve after a two-week adjustment period on the drug.

Some negative opinions of AZT are voiced in the book *Good Intentions* by Russ Nussbaum and the widely circulated article "Sins of Omission" (by Celia Farber, originally published in *Spin,* November 1989), which deals with the flaws in the research process that ultimately resulted in government approval of AZT.

There is no question that AZT is a toxic medication. But there is also no question that AZT is a useful antiviral that can stop the progression of HIV and significantly boost T4 cells. I personally believe that AZT is often overused. An important aspect of the decision-making surrounding AZT has to do with knowing when to use it and when to end the therapy.

Bernard Bihari, M.D., in an article for *BETA* magazine (November 1991), stated, "When AZT was first marketed for people with an AIDS diagnosis and/or fewer than 200 helper cells, I found that it was useful in two groups of patients. One was those who developed severe fatigue and weight loss, accompanied by fevers, night sweats, and other constitutional symptoms, without a causative opportunistic infection. . . . The other group of patients who frequently benefited from AZT were those who developed signs of HIV encephalopathy [memory loss, or dementia]." My clinical observations have been similar to Dr. Bihari's.

AZT was first approved for people with fewer than 200 T_4 cells. After additional studies, AZT was approved for early intervention in HIV infection or when T_4 cells went to 500 or below. The studies showed that in people who took AZT at 500 T_4 cells, the progression to symptomatic HIV or AIDS symptoms was slower than in people with T_4 cells at the same level who did not take AZT. But the data did not show a difference in the survival rate of either group.

In addition, data exists that does *not* support the use of AZT as an early intervention for HIV infection. A study produced by the Department of Veterans Affairs cited no difference between people on AZT and those not on the drug. However, this study was flawed—subjects were taking 1,200 mg of AZT, a dose abandoned early on as too high and too toxic.

Another issue to be considered is AZT resistance. In 1989, Dr. B. A. Larder and colleagues reported in *Science* magazine that virus obtained from patients with AIDS or symptomatic HIV who had received AZT for periods of approximately six months or longer frequently had HIV isolates, which demonstrated resistance to AZT in research studies. Other studies continued to document AZT resistance; Table 10-1, which matches T_4-cell levels to percentages of patients with resistance to AZT, was published in GMHC's *Treatment Issues* (August 30, 1990). According to these results, the earlier the drug was administered, the longer it took for resistance to develop. But the chance of resistance exists even if T_4 cells are in the higher ranges.

To complicate matters, AZT is now being tested extensively in combination with ddI and ddC. Combining the drugs seems to hinder resistance and lengthen the period of the effectiveness

TABLE 10-1.   AZT Resistance

Baseline T4-Cell Count	Percentage of Resistance After 12 Months on AZT
Less than 100	63–99 percent resistance
100–400	18–75 percent resistance
More than 400	11–59 percent resistance

of these nucleoside analogues (a type of antiviral that includes AZT, ddI, ddC, and D4T). But the toxicity of AZT is often unbearable to patients, and many people discontinue the drug for this reason.

How is it possible to find a way through this confusion in trying to decide whether or not to use AZT?

In my clinical experience, I have come up with the following guidelines for the patients I consult with:

• AZT alone or in combination with ddI or ddC is an extremely effective antiviral option.

• If you have never been on a nucleoside analogue and you're taking AZT for the first time, you will probably get the best results and the greatest increase in T4-cell counts.

• Taking into account the possibility that the natural antiviral options described in Chapter 8 might work, I hold off on using AZT, ddI, or ddC for people whose T4 cells are above or around 500.

• If T4 cells are consistently declining to between 200 and 300 or less, despite the use of a few different natural interventions, I recommend a combination of AZT and ddI or AZT and ddC in the hopes of stopping viral progression and giving the person in most cases a significant rise in T4 cells. This T4-cell rise can take a client out of the range where OIs manifest more frequently and to a point where other natural interventions can be tried to test their effect in maintaining the increase. I can best explain this approach with an anecdote.

Frank's T4 count had been steadily decreasing even though we had put together a natural-treatment regimen. This regimen had not been in place for long, and probably did not have enough time to work, since natural interventions take longer than the more aggressive treatments AZT, ddI, and ddC. But Frank's T cells fell to a point at which I considered an aggressive intervention to be necessary. I gave him all the information on all the options, and along with his health-care provider he chose to start AZT. Since the question of resistance consistently arises and long-term use of AZT might cause toxicity problems we are not yet aware of, Frank and I decided the intervention would be short-term, lasting only until his T4 cells significantly increased. Frank started with a count of 330, and within three months his T4 cells had jumped to 534. We reviewed all of his bloodwork and decided to take him off the AZT, adding an immune modulator, Tagamet, along with blue-green algae, in the hopes that these interventions would hold the rise Frank gained during AZT therapy and quite possibly continue the T4-cell increase. Once Frank made this change, his T cells went to 434, where they stayed for a while. Then they rose continuously to 700 over a year's time.

In Frank's case, the pieces all fell into place. From my point of view, long-term use of AZT risks not only a resistance problem but also potential toxicities to the body. As Dr. Bernard Bihari states in his *BETA* article, "Unfortunately, the antiviral agents currently available, the nucleoside analogues, AZT, ddI, and ddC, are toxic to many patients, have a limited timespan of activity because of the tendency of HIV to develop resistance to this class of drugs, and finally, may have limited long-term value because of their potential carcinogenicity." The carcinogenic effects of AZT have not been fully studied or documented.

In Frank's case, the T4 cells quickly rose to a safety zone in which we could try natural therapies again. Also, the AZT bought us the time to see if natural therapies he hadn't tried might now help to stabilize him. But in other cases, and especially where T4-cell counts are below 200, long-term use of AZT, ddI, and ddC is an option used often, and it's important to remain open to that possibility.

• The best scenario, then, is to wait until these antiviral drugs are absolutely necessary and then to use them for only a short period to boost the T4 cells back up to a point where natural interventions can be more effective.

• If T4 cells have already declined below 200 and these drugs have not boosted them into the safety zone above 350, continued use of these therapies might be the most beneficial approach.

• I still suggest using natural therapies to back up these interventions in the hope that together they can produce better results.

• Natural interventions—i.e., acupuncture and blue-green

algae—also help reduce the side effects and toxicity of nucleoside analogues.

• Consider combining AZT and ddI or ddC, since resistance is less likely and benefit is greater.

• If your T4 cells are dropping, and the natural therapies are not preventing further decline, do not wait. Intercede with the nucleoside analogues when T4 cells are between 250 and 400. Probably the earlier you intercede the better.

For a long time, my clients' doctors might say, "Why go off the AZT if it's working for you?" It was a constant uphill battle to convince them to acknowledge my reasoning. But at the 1992 Eighth International AIDS Conference, one of the abstracts of study results described a comparison of intermittent and continuous AZT treatment (PoB 3669). In this study, one group was on 500 mg of AZT daily and one on 500 mg of AZT four weeks on and four weeks off. The results showed that "intermittent AZT regimen is a practical way of administration. Interim results show a trend towards fewer severe anemia and a slower progression to AIDS, as compared to continuous therapy." The study continues, and I eagerly await the results, since this is consistent with the regimen I have been endorsing for the last two years. I go one step further: if your bloodwork changes for the better, discontinue the AZT and try to maintain T4-cell rises with less toxic substances. If HIV infection begins progressing again, as evidenced by T4-cell decrease and rises in beta-2 or neopterin levels, then another short-term AZT intervention would probably be beneficial.

Taking into consideration the information on AZT resistance, if you have been on AZT for a period and see T4-cell counts continually declining, I would suggest discontinuing the AZT and starting another antiviral therapy (ddI). This is another suggestion I have been giving people for the last two years. Recently, a study on ddI showed that patients who had changed to ddI early, as soon as AZT seemed to have lost effectiveness, did much better than patients who continued on the AZT. According to an oral preparation of the 14th AIDS Clinical Trials Group (ACTG), a federal research agency based in Washington, D.C., participants who were switched to 500 milligrams of ddI after being on AZT developed fewer AIDS-related infections and had modestly better T4 levels than those who remained on AZT.

As for the dosage of AZT alone, according to the most recent research as reported in an abstract at the Eighth International AIDS Conference 1992 (PoB 3724), the most effective dose of AZT is

- 500 mg daily.

To quote the study, "500 mg a day, even if presenting a higher number of side effects, appears the dosage of choice."

There was a report that 300 mg daily was just as effective, but later reports showed that 300 mg works okay early on, but that overall 500 mg is more effective for more progressed HIV and actually even as an early intervention as well.

THE LATEST ON NUCLEOSIDE ANALOGUES: VIDEX OR ddI (DIDEOXYINOSINE); HIVID OR ddC (DIDEOXYCYTIDINE)

If you've never taken AZT, ddI, or ddC, it appears that the best such treatment to start with is a combination of AZT and ddC, or AZT and ddI. These combinations have been studied and have shown greater effectiveness, better toleration, and less resistance than any one of these three drugs alone.

If you are deciding on one nucleoside analogue to start with, AZT and ddI are comparable for use by themselves but ddC alone does not look as effective. If you are currently on AZT and your T4 cells are dropping, it is becoming standard practice to stop the AZT and replace it with ddI, or to add ddI along with AZT, a practice I am uncertain about. One report on AZT resistance stated that after six months, viral resistance to AZT diminished. But one European study showed that this was not true for four out of the study's thirteen patients, so the results on resistance reversal are not yet definitive.

The doses that have been tested vary. As I said, for AZT, several studies showed 500 mg daily to be more effective than the 300 mg daily dose. Studies of combination antivirals have used AZT doses of 300 mg daily and ddI of 250 mg daily as well as 300 mg of AZT with .03mg/kg of ddC daily. (A / followed by "kg" refers to the body weight—in this case, .03 milligram per kilogram of body weight.)

To determine your dosage with this formula,

• divide your body weight by 2.2 to get your weight in kilograms; then multiply it by the milligrams—in this case .03. The product is your dose.

With most drugs, the starting dose is adjusted by body weight. Generally effective doses are only arrived at after years of research, and most drugs that have been approved for HIV testing were licensed by the FDA in the early stages of drug trials.

Usually, low doses of AZT and ddI are used for people on combination therapies, but you might want to try raising the dose if you are not reaching your intended goal. Starting with the lower dose and then working your way up to a higher dose gives your body a chance to adjust to this aggressive medication. In addition, if you are beginning combination therapy, add one drug at a time to isolate the cause of any side effects or toxicity if they occur.

In the case of AZT alone, the best starting dose is definitely 500. For ddI alone, there is not enough information available now for us to determine the best possible starting dose.

One serious side effect of ddI is pancreatitis, or inflammation of the pancreas. You can monitor for pancreatic irregularity by having your amylase levels taken regularly once a week for four weeks, starting seven days from the initial dose. If levels are not high during this adjustment period, you can go back to watching your amylase levels in your regularly scheduled bloodwork. Note that in a small Belgian study, ddI at 67 mg twice daily was compared to 250 mg twice daily, and there were no significant differences in effectiveness—T4-cell count elevations were seen in both groups, but a trend toward less pancreatitis was seen in the lower-dose group.

The doctors with whom I maintain a personal relationship—Paul Bellman, M.D., and Barbara Zeller, M.D.—are both prescribing between 200 and 400 mg daily of ddI in two doses according to body weight; these doses remain the same when using ddI in combination with AZT.

• People under 125 pounds use the 200-mg dose;
• people who are 125–190 pounds use the 300-mg dose;
• and people above 190 pounds use the 400-mg dose.

DdI comes in a pill form that is given in several different doses, and in a powdered form. In order to get enough buffer in the stomach to digest the ddI with the right pH balance, it is important to take

• two pills twice a day. For example, if you are on 100 mg twice daily, two 50-mg pills twice daily would be the best way to take this drug.

Some doctors and pharmacists have argued with me, saying that they have never heard of giving ddI this way, in two pills. One person even called this method poppycock. But when I pulled out the bottle and showed him the manufacturer's instructions right on the label, this fellow stopped his laughing and name-calling. (DdI will soon be available in orange flavor. With the powdered form, there is enough in the package to create the correct pH balance.)

The other major side effect of ddI and ddC is peripheral neuropathy, pain and tingling in the extremities and joints, usually of the hands and feet. Many people who are HIV+ are diagnosed with peripheral neuropathy even prior to starting ddI and ddC, and people with this preexisting condition often have trouble taking these drugs because they exacerbate it. I discuss peripheral neuropathy in Chapter 13, OI Treatments.

COMBINATION THERAPIES

DdC is a drug approved by the FDA for combination therapy only—that is, it is approved for prescription use only with AZT. Here's the reason why.

Early laboratory testing of ddC showed this substance to have been remarkably effective against HIV, but in human testing the side effects were so severe that it was impossible to administer it in the dosages associated with this anti-HIV reaction. However, the drug company Hoffmann-La Roche combined ddC and AZT, and this combination proved effective.

The rationale behind this method, called combination therapy, was to try to eliminate AZT resistance by administering an additional antiviral with it. Since ddC and AZT both work on the enzyme reverse transcriptase (RT), though at different points, the idea was that if you weren't able to intercept RT "coming in the front door" you would get it "going out the back." It was an attractive idea and a convenient one. And combination therapy actually works quite well.

Although approved for combination with AZT, ddC is *never* used in combination with ddI, since the drugs have similar toxicity and side effects. But another form of combination therapy pairs AZT with ddI. Studies have shown that both the AZT/ddC combination and the AZT/ddI combination have a synergistic effect, meaning that the effect of both together is greater than the combined total of each drug administered separately. However, ddC is not as effective as AZT or ddI alone, and is not approved as a therapy on its own (called monotherapy).

Regarding the method of combining the drugs, research to date shows that administering the drugs simultaneously rather than on an alternating basis is the superior method.

When compared with monotherapy, the benefits from combination therapy include:

- fewer resistant mutations of HIV after the same period on monotherapy
- larger T_4-cell-count increases
- stabilized increases over a longer period of time
- a greater reduction in opportunistic infections

As I stated earlier, I recommend combination treatments for three- to six-month periods, since the greatest T_4-cell increases occur over a short period. Both AZT/ddI and AZT/ddC are effective, but in my experience the AZT/ddC combination gives a greater initial T_4-cell increase than does AZT/ddI. T_4-cell increases on AZT/ddI are comparable, but they take longer to develop. If you decide on long-term combination therapy, AZT/ddI is probably the best choice as there is considerable data to support long-term stabilization of T_4 cells. If you wish to return to the more natural therapies but give your T_4 cells a boost before you do so, it is my experience that the AZT/ddI combination gives the best results in the shortest period of time.

With regard to dosage, I will give the standard recommendations here, but you must consult your doctor on this as well. Remember, dosages for most drugs are figured initially according to body weight, so if you are a small person it is likely that you can get the same results from a smaller dose than those suggested here.

Before I cite the recommended dosages, you should understand that although you take both drugs simultaneously in combination therapy, you need to begin the course with one week of one drug alone so you can isolate the causes of any possible side effects.

DdI comes in powder and chewable tablets. To maximize absorption of chewable tablets of ddI, take two tablets at a time on an empty stomach. With the powder, which appears to be easier to tolerate, only one packet at a time is necessary for proper absorption.

The powder form of ddI comes in doses of 100 mg, 167 mg, 250 mg, and 375 mg. The chewable tablets are available in doses of 25 mg, 50 mg, 100 mg, and 150 mg. There is also a powder available in pediatric doses.

DdC comes in two doses—.375-mg and .75-mg capsules and a syrup that is 50 mg per teaspoon.

AZT is available in 100-mg capsules and a syrup that is 50 mg per teaspoon.

The prescribed dosages of combination therapies vary greatly. I base my recommendations below on reading studies and articles, clinical observations, and the results of a study reported at the Eighth International AIDS Conference (PoB 3724), which showed the 500-mg dose of AZT to be more effective than the 300-mg dose.

These are the dosages I recommend:

• For AZT/ddI combination therapy, 500 mg of AZT with 200 mg of ddI.
• For AZT/ddC combination therapy, 500 mg of AZT with 2.25 mg of ddC.
• The AZT should be administered in five doses spread evenly throughout the day (but a middle-of-the-night dose is not necessary).
• The ddI should be taken in two 100-mg doses—one with the first AZT dose of the day and one with the last dose in the evening.
• The ddC should be taken in three .75-mg doses—with the first, third, and last dose of AZT. There is no need to take a dose in the middle of the night.

SUMMARY: AZT, ddI, ddC—THE NUCLEOSIDE ANALOGUES

I encourage people to do as much reading as they can on products before they begin taking them, and to follow the recommendations outlined in Chapter 5 on monitoring their bloodwork. In addition to that, in a very general sense, I recommend AZT and ddI or AZT and ddC to people who have consistent T4-cell decreases and other supporting bloodwork deficiencies and who have T4-cell counts between 250 and 400 after several decreases. Once they begin the drugs, I monitor them until their T4 cells rise to above 400 or 500 and then discontinue the nucleoside analogues. But I support the T4-cell increase with aggressive immune modulators and one or two alternative therapies as well. In most cases, the increased T4-cell count is maintained or drops slightly and then begins increasing again.

As usual, I am adamant about the importance, when you are on these treatment regimens, of following your bloodwork and making decisions based on sound medical observations. In addition, check with your doctor about monitoring bloodwork for toxicity from these drugs. Because AZT can cause RBC and WBC depletions, when it was first approved, doctors gave weekly CBC tests (see Chapter 5) for four weeks to make sure patients were not experiencing this toxicity. And with ddI amylase levels were taken on the same schedule to monitor any pancreatic problems. Many practitioners have slackened on these precautionary measures. I believe they are still beneficial.

COMPOUND Q OR GLQ223 (TRICOSANTHIN)

As a treatment for HIV infection and AIDS, Compound Q (not yet FDA-approved) has been in use since the end of 1988. At that time a report appeared that a drug produced from the Chinese cucumber, also known as tricosanthin, selectively killed the HIV virus in the test tube. Unfortunately, when patients themselves tried this—people who had no idea of proper use, possible side effects, or how to reduce the side effects—a death occurred that seemed to be linked to the use of the compound. Since that time, testing and experience have resulted in guidelines for the proper use of this therapy, and Compound Q has emerged as one of the important antiviral choices for the management of HIV infection.

A clinical update in *PI Perspectives* (April 1992) reported, "Of the limited number of experimental anti-HIV compounds which employ mechanisms different from AZT, GLQ223 is furthest along in clinical trials, testing safety and efficacy." These trials look promising, providing new hope for this drug's effectiveness.

One study (PoB 3442) of GLQ223 in patients with AIDS linked dosages of Compound Q to positive changes in bloodwork. When the initial death occurred, the fear of another such incident led practitioners to lower the dose to such a small amount that only 25 percent of the people taking the drug seemed to experience benefits, including T_4-cell rises. But drug companies and community-based organizations have continued to run studies on this drug, and at least three telling studies exist. As a result, we now have the information on how to infuse higher doses and to increase the number of people who experience significant T_4-cell increases.

Compound Q must be administered under the supervision of people who have had experience with it. The patient who died while using Compound Q died because the substance was administered incorrectly. If you decide to use this treatment option, it must be administered by people who

- have experience with the drug
- understand the drug
- currently have patients on the drug
- routinely monitor patients several days after the drug is infused

If you are interested, you will find reliable sources for researching this drug listed in the Resource Guide.

Matt Powell, writing in the *PWA Newsline*, reports that Ellen Cooper of the FDA has explicitly stated that Compound Q "must be administered under the auspices of an M.D." But Powell goes on to assert that critical-care nurses or nurse practitioners can effectively administer Compound Q as long as they have had experience with the drug.

Most patients are started at a low dose that is built up slowly to prevent side effects. During the initial infusions, side effects that occur for one to five days after infusion and then resolve, usually include

- two to five days of muscle aches and pain;
- fevers, generally ranging from between 100 and 101 degrees Fahrenheit;
- and itching or rashes.

Matt Powell states that you can avoid these side effects to some degree with Benadryl and other over-the-counter medications. The people who administer the drug should inform you of how to deal with possible side effects.

Compound Q seems to be relatively inexpensive, and it is obtainable through buyers clubs without a prescription. It is administered by an IV drip and is usually given to groups of ten to fifteen people, all monitored by licensed medical staff. Compound Q has been used on at least 3,000 HIV+ people and has been proven safe with AZT and ddI in studies by Gene Labs and Project Inform.

In the latest study, reported in Amsterdam, patients received dosages of 36 to 50 mg/kg of body weight. As I explained before, to determine the correct dosage,

- divide your weight by 2.2 (to get your weight in kilograms);
- multiply the quotient by mg of the drug—in this case, 36 or 50.

The doses, which seem to be safe when escalated over a period of time, go as high as

- 100 mg/kg

and new significant T4-cell rises have been seen at the higher doses, even after forty weeks of treatment with the lower doses and no previous T4-cell increases. Seventy-five percent of the people using the compound seemed to have either T4-cell increases or stabilization.

I have only skimmed the surface here of the information available on this drug. Project Inform, listed in the Resource Guide, is probably your best source of information on Compound Q, because the organization is responsible for some of the Phase I trials on the drug.

I recommend this drug for patients who do not stabilize on nucleoside analogues—that is, who are on AZT or ddI and have consistently decreasing T4-cell counts—and have T4-cell counts between 50 and 400. In the past, caregivers rarely administered Compound Q for patients with T4 cells below 50, but nowadays they do. It is my opinion that Compound Q will come of age, be FDA-approved, and become widely used, but you can never tell what's going to happen. Unfortunately, FDA approval is very difficult to come by for small, community-based studies of drugs that are not backed by large drug companies. Compound Q seems to be safe in combination with AZT, ddI, or ddC.

PEPTIDE T

Peptide T, a string of amino acids, was developed at the National Institute of Mental Health in 1986. In 1988–89, a Phase I trial of this treatment for HIV infection was completed in Boston, and these were the results:

- T-cell-count stabilization
- significant reversal of HIV-related neurocognitive disorders, such as dementia and peripheral neuropathy

I believe that Peptide T, not yet FDA-approved, should have been on the market a long time ago. This basically nontoxic string of amino acids shows much promise, not only as a treatment for dementia and peripheral neuropathy but also as an antiviral. Peptide T works by blocking the CD4 receptor sites that the virus latches on to just before it infects a cell.

Peptide T is readily available (and currently, *only* available) through buyers clubs and is certainly an option for HIV infection, and no prescription is needed for purchase. In my experience, Peptide T works best for people with peripheral neuropathy (tingling or numbness in the hands and feet) or with dementia or short-term memory loss.

Peptide T is available in two different forms:

- as a liquid that is administered intranasally or inhaled
- as a subcutaneous (under the skin) injection

I usually recommend the injectable preparation only for people who have severely damaged sinuses.

Only one case of toxicity has been reported in the literature with regard to Peptide T; that person developed a rash. Some report an irritation of the sinuses, since the drug is in an alcoholic solution. Information on Peptide T is readily available, the treatment is listed in the AmFAR treatment directory, and a Phase II clinical trial of Peptide T is currently under way, which might put this drug on the market very soon. In the meantime, people with peripheral neuropathy can try to join the trial (call 1-800-TRIALS-A for information) or secure it from a buyers club (listed in the Resource Guide).

T4-cell count is not relevant with respect to Peptide T. However, since this is a drug, if T cells are above 500, I usually avoid using Peptide T until other treatment options have been exhausted.

TRENTAL (PENTOXIFYLLINE)

Trental is a prescription drug that has been used worldwide for more than a decade in the treatment of circulatory problems, for which it is FDA-approved. In laboratory tests, this drug has been shown to decrease TNF (tumor necrosis factor) levels as well as HIV activity. Excessive levels of TNF have also been linked to wasting syndrome (see section on triglycerides, Chapter 5).

Initially, I intended to describe this drug in Chapter 15, Nutrition and HIV, since the results of early studies showed significant improvement in people with wasting syndrome. But later studies, one by the AIDS Clinical Trials Group (ACTG) and others reported at the 1992 Eighth International AIDS Conference, also showed that

• 400 mg three times daily of Trental has some antiviral capability. In one study, HIV titers, a measurement of the amount of HIV in one's system, dropped to below one tenth of pretreatment levels. Since this drug is relatively nontoxic, I recommend it if T cells are consistently falling and have gone below 500, or if triglyceride levels are climbing and go above 200. The drug has been tested on people with T4 cells under 200 as well. (Recent drug trials doubled the 400-mg dose; at this higher dosage, there were reports of side effects—including vision and skin problems. Make sure you are monitored closely for side effects of any prescription drug.)

Elevated triglyceride levels are a sign of excessive TNF activity, and therefore decreased triglyceride levels after treatment with Trental would be a sign of efficacy. This was significantly demonstrated in the data from the Amsterdam conference study.

Another interesting aspect of Trental is that it is not a nucleoside analogue and does not work the way AZT does. Therefore, it might enhance and work well with nucleoside analogues. As a matter of fact, one study presented at the Amsterdam conference showed that Trental enhanced the activity of ddI in laboratory tests (PoA 2326). Since increased TNF levels seemed to completely reverse the antiretroviral effect of AZT and ddC, Trental, possibly by reducing TNF, increased the effect of AZT and ddC. So Trental, by reducing TNF, probably improves absorption, which in turn increases the efficacy of other medications.

Trental is recommended for use in combinations with AZT, ddC, or ddI, or possibly prior to the use of nucleoside analogues as a less toxic antiviral therapy. It is easily available by prescription. Trental's way of working is similar to—though much more aggressive than—that of the nontoxic therapy NAC, discussed in Chapter 8.

D4T (STAVUDINE)

At the Amsterdam conference there were at least four reports of studies of D4T conducted in different parts of the United States (PoB 3011, 3016, 3022, 3023, 3027, 3029, 3030, 3033). D4T is a nucleoside analogue that blocks reverse transcriptase but is less toxic and more effective than the current therapies. D4T yielded both longer-term T4-cell increases and lowered toxicity. This drug, not yet FDA-approved but currently in Phase II studies, will soon be readily available. Those who have not responded to AZT or ddI can secure D4T through an expanded-access program by calling the Bristol-Myers Squibb Company at 1-800-842-8036. Your doctor must complete some paperwork first; then the drug company will supply D4T free of charge, and you will become part of the study results.

The dose that was cited as most effective was

• 2 mg/kg of body weight daily.

This drug has been widely studied, and its development is heavily financed by a drug company, so FDA approval is right around the corner.

CONCLUSION

There is no doubt that an antiviral regimen is an extremely important part of an HIV treatment regimen. Theoretically, an antiviral combined with an immune-modulating treatment should be able to stop HIV progression and rebuild a person's immune system. Remember, used effectively, the most toxic therapies can be a stepping-stone to long-term use of the less toxic therapies. The more toxic the drug, the shorter the period in which you will want to use it.

Starting with the least toxic antivirals, mentioned in Chapter 8, monitor your bloodwork and methodically review the efficacy of each antiviral until you see a positive effect, saving the most toxic therapies for later. For people with T cells below 200, a short period on nucleoside analogues—AZT, ddI, and ddC—can often boost T cells to a point at which less toxic therapies and immune modulators work more effectively and can serve as a treatment regimen to replace the toxic nucleoside analogues.

The most important part of an effective treatment regimen is your belief in that regimen. If you decide on AZT, believe that it will work for you, and believe you will not experience side effects, you will probably reduce the intensity of side effects. I'm not urging you to deny the possibilities that the treatment might not benefit you or might be toxic to you. Instead, I'm urging you to *acknowledge* the possibilities but *believe* in the most positive outcomes. Your belief is your most powerful weapon:

• believe in your health;
• believe in your will to live;
• and believe in the effectiveness of the treatment or treatments you choose.

CHAPTER 11

Special Concerns of Women

Over the course of the HIV pandemic, the battle against stereotypes has never let up. From the start, HIV infection was characterized as "the gay men's disease," and it took far longer than it should have for people inside and outside of the HIV community to recognize the infection in other groups. For women, that recognition is still to come. In the realms of research, treatment, and health-care policymaking, HIV+ women and the concerns specific to them have been excluded. The damage to infected women has been and continues to be great, and our health-care system is still far—very far—from correcting this shameful situation.

The special issues involving HIV+ women stem from these two facts:

- There are important differences between how HIV manifests itself in women and how it is expressed in men.
- There are important differences between how the health-care establishment treats women and how it treats men.

As a result, women have been and are still dying from HIV infection even before they are diagnosed with AIDS.

In this chapter, I attempt to unravel the tangles of information and *mis*information that have blocked the flow of knowledge and care to women with HIV infection. This means clarifying issues in three separate areas:

- diagnosis
- health-care access
- research

THE SPECIAL CARE WOMEN REQUIRE

Women infected with HIV often become symptomatic and even die without ever having been diagnosed with AIDS. The reasons for this are much more social or political than medical:

• As more than one observer has pointed out, in our health-care system, HIV+ women are seen as *carriers* of the virus to men and children rather than as people requiring care.

• Most early signs of HIV infection in women involve the reproductive tract and are treated as isolated gynecological complaints. Although most women see gynecologists or medical caregivers in public health clinics for their medical care, in general these personnel are untrained and remain unaware that HIV frequently manifests itself in the following ways in women:

- chronic vaginal infections
- chronic pelvic infections
- chronic pelvic pain
- menstrual changes, irregularities, cessations, or problems
- bacterial pneumonias and other respiratory problems
- abnormal Pap smears
- cancer of the cervix, vagina, and vulva
- blood disorders such as anemia and thrombocytopenia
- wasting
- any sexually transmitted disease—such as syphilis, gonorrhea, genital warts, herpes, or chlamydia

Regarding the last entry on the list, HIV+ women experience sexually transmitted diseases (STDs) more frequently and have more complications from them than men do. Because studies of HIV infection in women are nearly nonexistent, the reasons for these increases are controversial: some argue that STDs and other gynecological disorders are cofactors in infection, while others point out that the sores involved in these conditions could play a role in transmission.

For a detailed description of the symptoms of HIV infection that are specific to women, see Table 4-2 at the end of Chapter 4.

THE GOVERNMENT'S ROLE

Although many gynecologists and clinic personnel may be ignorant of the signs and symptoms of HIV infection in women, the negligence doesn't stop with the medical establishment. As I explained in Chapter 4, the federal government created a definition of AIDS as a way of deciding who would receive federal disability benefits. In 1982, the Centers for Disease Control and Prevention (CDC) came up with a list of life-threatening conditions resulting from immune suppression that would indicate a diagnosis of AIDS. Those who had one or more conditions on the list had AIDS; those who didn't match the list didn't have the disease—and those who didn't have AIDS didn't get benefits.

Needless to say, *none* of the symptoms of HIV infection specific to women made it onto the CDC's original list because all the original research was done with men. As a result, HIV+ women have been underdiagnosed and undertreated for the infection; the lack of clear diagnoses could prevent them from receiving life-saving prophylactic treatment against recurring opportunistic infections. In 1991, following years of activism, the CDC proposed to change its definition of AIDS to include T4-cell counts under 200, but the agency still excluded from its definition the conditions specific to women. The CDC added invasive cervical cancer to the definition of AIDS in January 1993, but this seems to be a token to quiet the activists demanding change.

A final point about diagnosis: most women know, at least intuitively, that the health-care system treats their medical symptoms differently than it treats those of men. Find me a patient whose headaches, weight loss, or fatigue has been ascribed to "stress," and there's a high likelihood that that patient is a woman. If you are a woman reading this book, be aware of what you're up against and make peace with the fact that you must be your own advocate. A good friend of mine described having unbearable mood swings during menstruation. Her doctors constantly tried to placate her, suggesting the trouble was all in her mind. Finally, though, she found a woman gynecologist who began treatment for hormonal imbalance and her symptoms resolved. Living in fear of your doctor only allows errors like this to continue. Here are some guidelines for asserting yourself in the face of medical caregivers who might doubt or dismiss your reports of your medical situation:

• Don't let anybody pat you on the head and send you away.
• Keep talking until somebody listens—and keep searching until you find a health-care team that knows what it's doing.
• Don't ignore low-grade infections just because they're familiar. Realize that vaginal infections can be a sign of lowered resistance brought about by immune suppression—and untreated vaginitis can itself stress an already compromised immune system.
• Stay one step ahead: read, read, read, to educate yourself on the symptoms of HIV and on the blind spots in the outside world that you are likely to encounter.
• Don't stop with *medical* treatment. Like every other condition, gynecologic symptoms respond well to holistic and natural treatments and a wealth of effective options exist. Seek out the natural and dietary alternatives, attend support groups specifically for (or at least including) HIV+ women, and collect information from the other women's experiences. Love and empower yourself.

HIV AND PREGNANCY

A special issue of *PWA Newsline* (October 1990) made the point outright: "Once a positive woman is pregnant (or any woman, really) the focus is entirely on the fetus." Very little research exists on pregnancy and HIV infection, but these points have been established:

• HIV+ women with no symptoms appear to have the same chances of achieving a healthy, full-term pregnancy and delivery as noninfected pregnant women do.
• In asymptomatic women, pregnancy does not appear to speed progression of HIV infection. Early researchers theorized that pregnancy would speed progression because it suppresses the mother's immune system to enable her to retain the fetus.

• In women with advanced HIV infection, full-term pregnancy may accelerate progression.

• Although all babies of HIV+ mothers are born with their mothers' immune systems so that they test HIV+, most test HIV− after developing their own immune systems (at age 18 months to two years). Current estimates suggest that 20–30 percent of these babies become infected and remain HIV+.

• HIV has been found in breast milk, and breast-feeding increases the risk of transmission from mother to baby.

TREATMENT ISSUES

Many of the most effective or promising drug treatments are available to HIV+ people only through clinical drug trials, and for anyone with the HIV infection, discovering and entering the appropriate drug trials is a major part of a well-rounded treatment program. But for women, the doors to the clinical trials they need have been from the beginning and still remain slammed shut. As reported in the February–March 1992 edition of the *Critical Path AIDS Project* newsletter,

• Of all the people enrolled in drug trials throughout the country, only 7 *percent* are women.

A federal research agency, the AIDS Clinical Trials Group (ACTG), has analyzed this tiny female portion of the total enrollees and has found that it breaks down this way:

• Most women in trials have had access to the antivirals AZT and ddI.

• The trials with the fewest women are those restricted to symptomatic HIV+ people.

• Although HIV infection is managed through the treatment of opportunistic infections as they arise, women's enrollment in OI drug trials is similarly restricted; in 1991, only 7.5 percent of their participants were females—even though it is well known that researchers who conduct trials for drugs that treat acute OIs *have trouble finding people to enroll*. The result is that opportunistic infections in women have gone unstudied.

In March 1992, the *Critical Path AIDS Project* magazine offered a list of recommendations (in an article by Iris Long, Ph.D.) for addressing women's HIV+ treatment issues, and many of them fit very well with the underlying theme of this book:

Don't wait for somebody else to do it; do it yourself.

But Dr. Long's guidelines speak to the federal decision-makers as well as HIV-infected women. I end this chapter with these recommendations in the hope that health-care workers and researchers will see them as a call to arms and that my female readers will see them as concrete steps toward finding and receiving thorough, effective care:

• *All* drugs under study should be analyzed for their effects on women, and disseminating these findings to medical personnel should be a top priority.

• I urge all HIV+ women to look into the Women's Interagency Health Study currently (*finally*) being launched by the CDC, the National Institute of Allergy and Infectious Diseases, and other federal agencies. If you get involved early, you and your caregivers and advocates could have a real effect on the design and implementation of this longitudinal study. Write to or call the Centers for Disease Control and Prevention in Atlanta for information (see the Resource Guide).

• Continue to pressure the CDC to redefine AIDS. The proposal to broaden the definition by adding T4-cell counts under 200, bacterial pneumonia, and cervical cancer is not enough. It appears that HIV+ women themselves need to educate the policymakers on how HIV infection manifests in women.

• It is imperative that clinical trials of drugs to treat acute opportunistic infections be designed to include women. Women activists and activists on behalf of women need to gain access to FDA decision-makers and pressure for the fundamental changes that will let women participate in these trials.

• Obstetricians, gynecologists, and other reproductive-health workers need to take an active role and *demand* the information they need to understand the relationship between women's bodies and HIV infection. Where that information is nonexistent, they need to raise the questions and *demand* that researchers design studies to come up with the answers.

A FINAL NOTE

I want to end with the caution with which I began this chapter:

- HIV manifests itself in women in specific ways that differ from manifestations in men,
- but women get all the infections men get as well.

If you are an HIV+ woman, don't let this be the single chapter you read. And when you read Chapter 4, on symptoms, make sure you read both Table 4-1 (HIV-Related Infections) *and* Table 4-2 (HIV-Related Symptoms in Women). Read this chapter, read the whole book, and then *read this chapter again.* You are your own best advocate. I hope you'll be inspired here to raise your voice and never let it fall until you get what you need and deserve.

CHAPTER 12

Putting It All Together:
Case Studies

To give you a clear picture of all the recommendations I've covered so far, in this chapter I sketch out twenty-one case studies drawn from my files and include charts of these clients' bloodwork and records of their treatments. Since we have discussed a holistic view—one that encompasses not only treatment interventions but also changes in life-style—I have chronicled treatment interventions as well as life changes. For instance, if a client started meditating, that would be one component in a complete treatment plan, and I include it in my case description.

When you study the bloodwork flowcharts that accompany these studies (each case study has a flowchart), you'll notice a discrepancy between them and the model flowchart I supply in Chapter 5 for helping you monitor your bloodwork. I chose the cases in this chapter from my files to illustrate how various individuals responded to treatment over a relatively long period of time. Since I wrote these case studies, the importance of triglyceride and albumin levels has surfaced, and I incorporated these readings into the Chapter 5 flowchart. The flowchart used in this chapter was designed before the new information emerged. Also, as reference ranges can vary from lab to lab (as I explained in Chapter 5), I've eliminated them to avoid confusion.

INTEGRATING YOUR APPROACHES TO HEALING

I recently heard Frank Lipman, an M.D. and licensed acupuncturist, explain his approach to integrating the many different aspects of healing. In the HIV+ person, combining these diverse efforts can significantly increase the quality of life. In the beginning, there might seem to be a lot to think through, but once your options are in place, you are likely to experience your treatment regimen itself as a fulfilling part of your life.

Fulfilling might be a difficult word for many newly diagnosed HIV+ people to digest, but it is not unusual to hear at a support group that "finding out I was HIV+ was the best thing that ever happened to me." As people search for the combination of services and options they wish to integrate into their healing processes, they often experience situations that stimulate personal, spiritual, and psychological growth. Dr. Lipman talked extensively of our thoughts and feelings around HIV, and how for many of his patients deeply buried emotions surface during acupuncture treatments. Louise Hay would say that these emotions are very possibly the *cause* of the illness—the very discoveries we need to make so that we may heal.

Inspired by Dr. Lipman's lecture, I put together a list of the separate issues that any person beginning a healing journey should address and combine. Together, these are the separate elements that could be integrated to form an effective treatment program for HIV infection:

1. Western mainstream medicines. These often toxic, very aggressive medications are frequently overlooked by "holistic practitioners." But *holistic* means "addressing the whole," and many of these medications are extremely beneficial in addressing and eliminating medical problems. Even when there is toxicity, benefits can outweigh adverse reactions. Knowing when to use these interventions and when not to is an integral part of a healing regimen.

2. *Alternative therapies.* This category of therapies, which includes Chinese herbology and homeopathic medicine, is often discounted by "Western practitioners," whose egos could stand to be deflated a bit. Often nontoxic and beneficial, these therapies

are as integral to a treatment regimen as are mainstream interventions.

3. Nutritional guidance. Food is the fuel that runs us. Unfortunately, many nutritional practitioners say they can cure HIV, and they prescribe so many supplements that the person becomes not only emotionally overloaded but the pills become a constant reminder that he or she is dealing with a life challenge, a situation the person often interprets as "I am ill." Equally disturbing is the tendency for an overly complex nutritional program to confuse matters: if you are taking twenty-five substances every day, it will be impossible to know what is working for you. The important thing, in seeking nutritional guidance, is to trust and believe in any practitioner you choose. For this reason, you'll need to do some diversified research to find the nutritional adviser who is right for you (see Chapter 15, Nutrition and HIV).

4. Bodywork. Acupuncture, chiropractic, and massage all fall into the category of bodywork. Relying on recommendations from other HIV+ people as well as your own personal instincts about the different practitioners you meet should easily secure you someone in this area you can trust. Some people choose to combine acupuncture and massage, any two of the three, or even all three. I encourage clients to try as many variations as possible and then to ask themselves

- which they are most comfortable with,
- which they believe in most,
- which gives them the most physical relief,
- which gives them the most emotional relief,
- and which yields labwork benefits.

I recommend it once or twice a week, but bodywork even every three to four weeks can be beneficial for maintenance in people with T4 cells above 500.

5. Stress reduction/spiritual journey. Meditation and stress reduction are clearly parts of the healing experience. Spiritual beliefs can include:

- centering
- meditating
- fear reduction
- praying

As I noted earlier, in Narcotics Anonymous they say, "Fear is lack of faith," always believing that God, a higher power, or whatever you choose to have faith in will give you no more than you can handle. Deep spiritual beliefs, guided visualization, affirmation, meditation, and the discovery of love within each person you meet will help you to achieve a quality of life and level of sanity that might be difficult to maintain otherwise. Exercise, bicycle riding, deep breathing, yoga, and other such activities also function to reduce stress. Sometimes, any activity that can refocus your mind on a joyful place rather than a place of worry will give you a moment's spiritual connection. Look at the trees and flowers or step outside and look up on a starry night and you will see what I mean. (See Chapter 17, The Mind–Body Connection: Psychoneuroimmunology, for more information.)

6. Emotional work. You may want to do this work with a psychotherapist or social worker—one, it is hoped, who does not rely on drugs or use a Freudian approach, but who will help you explore and deal with the emotions you experience daily. Louise Hay claims that her cancer was—literally *was*—the resentment of her father, who had abused her as a child. She had buried the memory of this abuse, and it only surfaced during the psychotherapeutic process. She described her tumor as her growing resentment of her father. When she forgave her father, her body's cancer began to shrink. She also incorporated in her treatment program all the aspects of healing listed above except Western medicine, though she does not speak out against the latter.

Working with a good therapist can greatly help you to reduce stress and achieve spiritual fulfillment. In fact, one part of *The Books: A Course in Miracles,* the spiritual path discussed by Marianne Williamson in her book *A Return to Love,* is a pamphlet that explores the similarities between spirituality and psychotherapy. According to *A Course in Miracles,* the two pursuits are identical, sharing the goal of getting the mind into perfect working order. *A Course in Miracles* holds that once the mind uncovers the blocks to the love within us, that love will be evident—and that love is God.

You might find one practitioner who is able to incorporate several of the aspects of the healing elements described above. You also may feel that some aspects are not for you. The bottom line is *results:* if you are having positive results, then whatever you are doing is the right combination. Sometimes results can also be measured in quality of life—although bloodwork and labwork are extremely important, to experience improvement in the quality of your life is to experience living proof that your program is working.

FORMULATING A TREATMENT PLAN

I encourage my patients and you, the reader, to use the flowchart in Chapter 5 to follow bloodwork and track lab results. If you study the chart, you'll see that it includes SGOT and SGPT, which are measurements of liver enzymes. These measurements will indicate prior liver damage, current hepatitis, and/or drug toxicity. In addition to these two measurements, two other markers on your bloodwork will indicate liver damage; they are the bilirubins, enzymes made by the liver. When all four markers are high, hepatitis is usually the explanation, but in my charting recommendations, only two are included.

When only the SGOT and SGPT rise, they might be indicating past liver damage or a chemical hepatitis caused by drugs, some of which are used in the treatment of HIV infection. When these liver enzymes rise, there are several possible responses:

- You can stop the drugs that are causing the damage. (Consult your physician before stopping the treatment.)
- You can take a natural substance that helps the liver metabolize toxic substances more readily, and thereby attempt to avoid further liver damage or bring liver enzymes down to normal.
- You can use aggressive mainstream liver-revitalizing agents.

The more natural substances that seem to bring down the liver enzymes are

- blue-green algae
- and thioctic acid (see Chapter 8).

Also, according to the company that distributes it, phyllmartin (an herb discussed in Chapter 8) cures hepatitis A, B, and C. Now, *cure* is a very hard word for me to swallow, and mainstream medicine denies that any cure currently exists for hepatitis. I have tried this herb on five clients, all of whom were diagnosed with chronic hepatitis; three had hepatitis A, one had hepatitis B, and one had hepatitis C. In three cases, the liver enzymes came down from counts of 500–800 to within the normal range, which is below 50. I am not sure whether the herb was entirely responsible, but three patients were not doing any other treatment that would have had this effect. Considering the low toxicity of phyllmartin in this case, I usually recommend this route to clients first.

Mainstream medical interventions for liver damage are alpha interferon and gamma globulin. Both of these substances have been tested with HIV infection, and both have yielded mixed results. But there is some evidence that these two drugs are also immune modulators. That might be a great benefit for people who are HIV+, since immune modulation is a necessary and integral component in any HIV treatment program.

Alpha interferon seems to be the least expensive of the two and the treatment of choice for most M.D.s. However, two articles, one in *PWA Newsline* (August 1992) and one in *Critical Path AIDS Project* (February 1992) magazine, have stated that alpha-interferon levels in people with T_4-cell counts below 500 might already be elevated, since the body is producing alpha interferon to fight off HIV. These articles hypothesize that raising the alpha interferon at this point might be without benefit. One article states that increased alpha-interferon levels have been associated with progression to AIDS. In three of my own clients on alpha interferon, I have noticed an expedited decline in T_4 cells when counts fall below 500, suggesting a connection.

Given this possibility, I have been recommending gamma globulin, even though it is more expensive. As I explained earlier, the cost is the only reason this treatment isn't prescribed more often. I have even heard stories of medical insurance carriers' pressuring against the further testing of gamma globulin for HIV+ people owing to the expense of the substance.

CASE STUDIES

If you do not understand your lab results, review Chapter 5 before reading the following case studies.

Note: I have chosen not to cover certain test results and treatment options in this chapter, owing to their newness at this writing. As I noted earlier, test results not covered here are triglyceride levels and albumin levels. Treatment options seldom used owing to recent developments are glycyrrhizin, bitter melon, Trental, and NAC.

Case 1: Dan

Dan, a thirty-four-year-old white male, came to me in May 1992. He had been on AZT for the preceding two years and had had a T4-cell count of 440 a year before I met him. By the time I first met him, his T4-cell count had dropped to 170. Dan meditated daily, saw a nutritionist, took tons of supplements recommended by the nutritionist, and was dealing with a booming career. I recommended that he stop the AZT and change to ddI, since such a long period on AZT usually results in AZT resistance. Such resistance was evidenced in Dan by the drop in his T4 cells. In addition to his 170 T4-cell count, his T4-cell percentage was 6—and 5 percent is the point at which extremely aggressive prophylaxis against at least five OIs is recommended.

Most people with 170 T4 cells have a higher percentage—a more usual reading would have been 10 or more percent. Dan's percentage reading was evidence of imbalance in his system, and this was further indicated by the CD4/CD8 ratio, which had gone from .24 to .09. Studies show that chances of infection increase when this ratio falls below .25.

Dan's liver enzymes—SGPT and SGOT—were elevated, and he had a history of alcohol consumption, which he had stopped a few years before. Elevations above 100 on these measurements suggest liver damage; if they are accompanied by high bilirubin measurements, hepatitis is a possibility.

In addition to recommending the change to ddI, I advised Dan to take the supplements blue-green algae and thioctic acid for the liver. As you can see in Figure 12-1, the T4-cell percentage, count, ratio, and the liver enzymes all showed the desired change. In addition, the beta-2 microglobulin had gone down .1 percentage point, not a great decrease but headed in the right direction, evidencing antiviral activity.

Also, the great rise in the T4-cell count and percentage took Dan out of the range in which many opportunistic infections are

FIGURE 12-1.   Dan (Case 1)

	6/22/91	5/92	8/18/92		
WBC	5.6	6.6	6.2		
RBC	3.6	3.3	4.4		
HGB	13.7	13.2	14.7		
HCT	40.8	38.6	43.6		
Triglycerides					
Albumin					
Platelets	203	195	224		
ESR or sed rate	9	/	/		
T$_4$ %	16	6	16		
T$_4$ #	440	170	350		
T$_8$ %	67	69	66		
T$_8$ #	1840	1960	1430		
CD$_4$/CD$_8$ ratio	.24	.09	.24		
Beta-2 micro-globulin	2.2	2.2	2.1		
P$_{24}$ antigen	.378		.419		
P$_{24}$ antibody	62		72		
Neopterin					
SGOT	54		37		
SGPT	88		65		

common. In this safety zone, I recommended immune modulation with Tagamet, naltrexone, and Antabuse, and a discontinuation of the ddI when the T4-cell count went above 400 and 20 percent. Notice that the T8-cell count is also high, above a thousand.

Case 2: Paula

Paula is a white female who works in a very stressful job. She is thirty-two years old. She contracted HIV through intravenous drug use and came to me in January 1991. Since her T4-cell count was 465 and her percentage was 52 percent, I saw no need to recommend AZT, as her doctor had. She was involved in a recovery process, but had not yet seriously incorporated stress reduction and other adjunct therapies.

Paula began a regimen of vitamin C, blue-green algae, and B_{12}. Over the next year, her T4 cells varied and the last entry, at the end of the year, showed more T4 cells than when she began. Even though her percentage declined, in this high range the change was insignificant. I considered this success—staying off AZT and maintaining this high level of T4 cells for a year. Who knows how much more time she will add to her asymptomatic period.

Case 3: John

John came to me in March 1992 when he had 29 T4 cells. He had never done any aggressive antiviral therapies (for example, AZT), and I recommended combination therapy of AZT/ddC. At that time there was more evidence in support of that combination; now I might recommend AZT/ddI, which is better for long-term stabilization. John also started acupuncture, and his T4 cells rose steadily to 187. His percentage is still low, as is his ratio, but to go from 29 to 187 T4 cells would strike most doctors as impossible. It is *not* impossible. It may be difficult, and the treatment regimen may need to be particularly aggressive, but I have seen at least thirty cases of T4 cells below 50 rising above 200. When John's T4-cell count reached 187, in July 1992, I recommended that he add naltrexone, Antabuse, and Tagamet to boost the T4 cells further. His T8 cells rose and his beta-2 fell. All these measurements demonstrate that this treatment regimen is working.

Case 4: Dennis

Dennis came in for a consultation in June 1991, after his T4 cells had dropped from 392 to 288. A forty-five-year-old black male, Dennis was extremely reluctant to follow his doctor's recommendation that he take AZT. He had read negative information about AZT and, although he did begin to take it a week before our meeting, he did not use it as prescribed. I suggested blue-green algae, Tagamet, Peptide T, vitamin E for dry skin patches (no more than 800 IU daily), lysine as a prophylaxis against herpes (a cofactor in HIV progression), and B_{12}. The results were an increase in T4-cell count of almost 200 points to 471, a T4-percentage rise to 31.4, and an increase in the CD4/CD8 ratio from .46 to .89, a considerable improvement.

After we jointly decided on this regimen, Dennis stopped taking the AZT and he informed his doctor of this decision. If the T4s had not gone up and continued to go down, I would have recommended an AZT/ddC combination, which works better over the short term. With a T4-cell count around 200, my aim is a quick increase, not long-term stabilization (which I would consider for T4s below 75). So, here is a case where AZT was not used and a significant rise was still seen.

Case 5: Tim

Tim is a forty-three-year-old white male who came in to see me in June 1991. His T4 cells were 669 and his liver enzymes were extremely elevated, above 200, indicating liver damage, possible hepatitis, and drug toxicity. He had been on AZT for a year and his T cells had risen from 500 to 669. He was concerned about the liver enzymes and was thinking of going on a more natural regimen and giving up the AZT. I supported this decision and helped him put together a treatment regimen consisting of Peptide T, blue-green algae, and vitamin B_{12}. For the next eight to nine months, his T4 cells decreased; in March 1992, they hit their low of 378. At that time, Tim was considering going back on AZT. I agreed with his decision to reconsider AZT therapy, but at the last minute he decided to wait one month and draw blood-work at that time. That was a very reasonable decision, since if the decline continued, it was important to intercede as soon as possible. But it did not—his T cells started to rise and continued to

FIGURE 12-2.   Paula (Case 2)

	1/31/91	4/19	9/5/91	12/3/91		
WBC	5.6	7.0	5.8	5.5		
RBC						
HGB	12.5	12.7	14.1	14.1		
HCT	38.4	37.0	41.3	40.4		
Triglycerides						
Albumin						
Platelets	92	62	71	71		
ESR or sed rate						
T4 %	52	44.0	46.0	43.0		
T4 #	465	583	655	552		
T8 %						
T8 #						
CD4/CD8 ratio	1.52	1.02	1.06	.93		
Beta-2 micro-globulin	2.60		2.50			
P24 antigen						
P24 antibody						
Neopterin						
SGOT						
SGPT						

FIGURE 12-3. John (Case 3)

	8/15/91	3/9/92	6/4/92	7/92			
WBC	4.4	2.93	3.40	3.55			
RBC	4.47	4.41	3.70				
HGB	12.6	12.2	10.8				
HCT	37.5	37.6	31.9				
Triglycerides							
Albumin							
Platelets	199	133	209				
ESR or sed rate		15	54				
T4 %	10	3	7	6			
T4 #	71	29	102	187			
T8 %	30	74		64			
T8 #	213	718		925			
CD4/CD8 ratio	.33	.04	.10	.09			
Beta-2 micro-globulin		3.5	2.5	2.3			
P24 antigen							
P24 antibody							
Neopterin							
SGOT	20	39	27				
SGPT	38	40	22				

FIGURE 12-4.   Dennis (Case 4)

	1/15/91	6/18/91	12/19/91		
WBC	3.3	2.5	3.2		
RBC	4.2	4.12	4.69		
HGB	13.1	13.5	14.6		
HCT	39.1	40.4	43.4		
Triglycerides					
Albumin					
Platelets	160	160	140		
ESR or sed rate	/	/	/		
T4 %	28.0	24.0	31.4		
T4 #	392	288	471		
T8 %					
T8 #					
CD4/CD8 ratio	.54	.46	.89		
Beta-2 micro-globulin	/	/	/		
P24 antigen					
P24 antibody					
Neopterin					
SGOT					
SGPT					

FIGURE 12-5. Tim (Case 5)

	6/91	12/91	2/92	3/92	4/92	6/92		
WBC	4.7	4.8	3.9	3.3	4.5	4.10		
RBC	5.05	4.96	4.46	4.24	3.91	3.81		
HGB	16.9	15.5	15.1	14.3	14.8	14.2		
HCT	48.1	43.6	42.8	40.9	40.7	39.2		
Triglycerides								
Albumin								
Platelets	253	225	209	272	278	187		
ESR or sed rate					26			
T_4 %	31.9	24.0		29.1	26	34		
T_4 #	669	432		378	447	518		
T_8 %	54.0	58.4		53.1	57.0	51		
T_8 #	1134	1051		690	980	777		
CD_4/CD_8 ratio	.59	.41		.54	.46	.66		
Beta-2 micro-globulin					2.9			
P_{24} antigen								
P_{24} antibody								
Neopterin								
SGOT	211		74		58	62		
SGPT	343		89		72	70		

rise, and he remains off AZT and stable with a T-cell count above 500. All along, his liver enzymes had been declining, owing partly to his discontinuing AZT and partly to the blue-green algae.

Case 6: Jane

This chart illustrates the variation from lab to lab in T4-cell count and other HIV-specific measurements. These two bloodworks were drawn at Smith-Kline Labs and National Health Laboratories a few days apart, and as you can see, there is a variation in T4-cell count of almost 100 points and 4 percent. In addition, there is a variation of .04 in the ratios and a drastic .7 difference in the two beta-2s. This comparison should illustrate for you the need to draw your bloodwork at the same lab all the time so you can rely on the accuracy of your result comparisons.

Case 7: Joaquin

Joaquin, a twenty-six-year-old Hispanic male, came to me in March 1992 when his T4 cells had dropped from 106 to 87. He had not been on any antivirals, but he was on Bactrim three times a week to prophylax against PCP. In addition, he had lost a lot of weight and was extremely thin. My recommendations included Trental, blue-green algae, an AZT/ddC combination, and Zovirax (800 mg/4 times daily). This aggressive regimen gave immediate results, and within two months his T cells were going back up. His beta-2 had also risen, which is a sign of viral activity, but in later bloodworks (not shown here) the beta-2 also began decreasing. When results are mixed, such as T cells rising and beta-2 cells rising, I recommend drawing blood more frequently, so that any additional action can be taken in a timely fashion.

Case 8: Bill

Bill first learned he was HIV+ in July 1990, when his T4 cells were 756. He was convinced there was nothing wrong and did not see the need for any intervention. Within a few months, his T cells had gone down only slightly, but he decided that he wanted to intercede early and maintain his health. I recommended vitamin C, blue-green algae, B₁₂, and acupuncture. On this regimen, his T4 cells continued to climb over the next year, and in October

FIGURE 12-6. Jane (Case 6)

	S.K. 6/92	N.H.L. 6/92			
WBC	5.2	5.2			
RBC	4.02	4.02			
HGB	12.5	12.1			
HCT	36.9	34.7			
Triglycerides					
Albumin					
Platelets	386	324			
ESR or sed rate	/	/			
T4 %	16	20			
T4 #	384	481			
T8 %	68	69			
T8 #	1632	1661			
CD4/CD8 ratio	.24	.29			
Beta-2 micro-globulin	2.8	2.1			
P24 antigen					
P24 antibody					
Neopterin					
SGOT	25	24			
SGPT	70	51			

FIGURE 12-7.   Joaquin (Case 7)

	10/21/91	3/31/92	5/5/92		
WBC	3.0	2.0	3.2		
RBC	3.3	4.2	3.79		
HGB	12.5	13.6	13.0		
HCT	37.9	41.6	36.8		
Triglycerides					
Albumin					
Platelets	158	93	94		
ESR or sed rate	/	/	30		
T4 %	9.3	8.5	10		
T4 #	106	87	120		
T8 %	73.2	78.2	75		
T8 #	834	798	900		
CD4/CD8 ratio	.13	.11	.13		
Beta-2 micro-globulin		3.06	3.3		
P24 antigen					
P24 antibody					
Neopterin					
SGOT					
SGPT					

FIGURE 12-8.   Bill (Case 8)

	7/23/90	10/25/90	1/22/91	4/2/91	7/9/91	10/3/91	1/7/92	3/26/92
WBC	9.3	8.6	7.6	8.5	8.9	8.2	8.6	7.9
RBC	5.25	5.01	5.17	4.88	4.98	4.89	5.09	5.31
HGB	15.9	15.1	15.7	14.9	15.7	15.3	15.5	16.3
HCT	48.3	45.2	47.4	44.2	45.5	46.8	46.7	48.5
Triglycerides								
Albumin								
Platelets	284	291	283	302	345	337	367	361
ESR or sed rate	1	1	0	3	0	1	26	8
T4 %	36.	33.7	36.5	/	41.5	39.9	42.5	38.8
T4 #	756	707	912	/	1120	1197	1105	1008
T8 %	38.6	42.1	38.3	/	38.1	36.4	34.4	33.8
T8 #	810	884	957	/	1028	1092	894	878
CD4/CD8 ratio	.93	.80	.95	/	1.08	1.09	1.23	1.14
Beta-2 micro-globulin	1.9	1.9	1.9	1.7	2.0	1.8	2.0	1.9
P24 antigen	/	/	/	/	/	/	/	/
P24 antibody	/	/	/	/	/	/	/	/
Neopterin	/	/	/	/	/	/	/	/
SGOT	15	14	15	14	20	33	22	17
SGPT	13	19	12	11	16	17	19	14

1991 they peaked at 1,197. They then began to decline again, and in March 1992 I recommended adding NAC to the regimen. After the next bloodwork, his T4 cells were stable again at 996. This is an example of two full years of life symptom free, with rising T cells and stable beta-2 cells with nontoxic treatments. By the way, Bill's doctor had recommended doing nothing until "your T cells get to 500. Then we'll put you on AZT." I'm glad Bill didn't wait.

Case 9: Ted

Ted had been on AZT for approximately two years, and his T4 cells had gone down from 500 to 218, when I first consulted with him in January 1992. He was drinking, and continues to drink, and relies totally on Western medical interventions. I recommended Zovirax (3 times daily) since he had a history of herpes, Bactrim (3 times weekly) since his T4 cells were below 20 percent, and a switch from AZT to ddI (300–400 mg daily). (The high dosage of ddI was recommended because Ted weighed approximately 200 pounds; most people would take between 200 and 300 mg of ddI.) Ted's T4 cells began rising, and they continue to show small, steady increases.

Case 10: Bob

Bob had been on AZT and his T cells were at 560 in June 1991, when I met him. A twenty-five-year-old Hispanic male, Bob was extremely interested in discontinuing AZT and starting a less toxic regimen that included Western medicine. I recommended Tagamet, naltrexone, Antabuse, blue-green algae, and vitamins C and B$_{12}$. In October, Bob's T4 cells were 882, and a count taken after that was 1,200. His percentage and ratio had gone down, but they bounced back on the next labwork. With an 882 T4-cell count, 17 is a low percentage, but the T4 cells are so high that the measurement compensates, even if the percentage and ratio are off. The best scenario is to have the percentage and ratio rise along with the T4-cell count itself.

Case 11: Sam

Sam was a twenty-two-year-old white male with a high-pressure administrative job. He was told to do nothing when he found out,

FIGURE 12-9.   Ted (Case 9)

	1/8/91	6/26/91	1/30/92	6/18/92		
WBC				6.1		
RBC				4.90		
HGB				14.9		
HCT				45.9		
Triglycerides						
Albumin						
Platelets				286		
ESR or sed rate	/	/	/	/		
T4 %	11.5	9.2	11.4	10.6		
T4 #	290	220	218	265		
T8 %	71.6	74.1	58.8	67.2		
T8 #	1816	1779	1124	1680		
CD4/CD8 ratio	.2	.1	.2	.2		
Beta-2 micro-globulin				2.20		
P24 antigen						
P24 antibody						
Neopterin						
SGOT	50					
SGPT	76					

Figure 12-10.   Bob (Case 10)

	6/18/91	10/30/91		
WBC	7.90	10.1		
RBC	4.72	4.90		
HGB	14.6	16.0		
HCT	47.7	47.9		
Triglycerides				
Albumin				
Platelets	223	314.0		
ESR or sed rate	/	/		
T4 %	25	17		
T4 #	560	882		
T8 %	55	60		
T8 #	1233	3114		
CD4/CD8 ratio	.45	.28		
Beta-2 micro-globulin	/	/		
P24 antigen	/	/		
P24 antibody	/	/		
Neopterin	/	/		
SGOT	/	/		
SGPT	/	/		

FIGURE 12-11.   Sam (Case 11)

	3/11/91	11/13/91	3/1/92	4/16/92	6/27/92		
WBC	/	5.57	6.5	6.86	8.7		
RBC	/	4.84	4.85	4.12	4.04		
HGB	/	14.9	15.2	13.3	12.7		
HCT	/	45.7	43.8	38.1	37.1		
Triglycerides							
Albumin							
Platelets	/	285	393	295	302		
ESR or sed rate	/	10	12	13	4		
T4 %	39	35	35	30	37		
T4 #	858	454	534	587	634		
T8 %	28	35	37	45	35		
T8 #	616	454	565	880	600		
CD4/CD8 ratio	1.39	1.00	.95	.67	1.00		
Beta-2 micro-globulin	/	1.6	2.0	1.8	1.5		
P24 antigen	/	66	129	142	183		
P24 antibody	/	20%	20%	38%	20%		
Neopterin							
SGOT					35		
SGPT					30		

in March 1991, that he was HIV+. At that time his T4 cells were
858. Six months later, when he had his next bloodwork (his
doctor let him go that long because his T4 cells were so high) the
reading was 454. This is an example of why, even if your T4 cells
are above 500, although some doctors would run lab tests every
six months, you should insist that your bloodwork be done every
three months. As this chart illustrates, your T4 cells could decline
by half during the period between tests—and you'd want to know
about any decline so that you might intercede early.

Sam's doctor did not choose to intercede with any toxic therapies. When his T4 cells were 454, his doctor still recommended
doing nothing. Sam was concerned, and arranged a consultation
with me. I understood his feelings regarding an all-natural regimen, and I recommended an herb treatment, blue-green algae,
B_{12}, vitamin C, and acupuncture. Sam was also doing meditation
and was involved in a twelve-step recovery program. His lab
results continued to rise. His beta-2 microglobulin count initially
went up, but this count usually takes a little longer to fall than the
other counts take to rise. Eventually, the beta-2 began its slow
descent.

Case 12: Gary

Gary is a forty-three-year-old black male who found out he was
HIV+ in June 1991 and immediately came to me for a consultation. He had contracted HIV from a prostitute. Initially, the
doctors told Gary to do nothing, because his T4-cell count was
616. Gary consulted with me at that time, and I recommended
blue-green algae, vitamin C, and B_{12}. Gary's T4 cells continued
to decline, so we modified his regimen in December of 1991,
adding Tagamet, naltrexone, and Antabuse. The bloodwork after that continued to rise, and in August 1992 his T4-cell count
was 769 and 23 percent. His liver enzymes were also rising, so
thioctic acid was added to the regimen and Tagamet was discontinued, since it can cause liver enzymes to rise.

Case 13: Sean

Sean was a twenty-five-year-old Los Angeles resident who had
contracted HIV while in college. For years his doctors told him to
do nothing, but when his T4 cells dropped to 360 they recom-

FIGURE 12-12.   Gary (Case 12)

	6/27/91	7/24/91	12/11/91	1/9/92	5/18/92	8/8/92		
WBC		6.70	10.8	7.00	7.4	7.4		
RBC		4.61	4.4	4.38	3.98			
HGB		14.2	13.2	13.0	12.2	13.2		
HCT		41.6	40.1	41.4	35.3	39.8		
Triglycerides								
Albumin								
Platelets		144		282	300	265		
ESR or sed rate								
T_4 %	17	20	17		23.90			
T_4 #		616	431	509	648	769		
T_8 %								
T_8 #								
CD_4/CD_8 ratio	.45	.47			.42			
Beta-2 micro-globulin								
P_{24} antigen								
P_{24} antibody								
Neopterin								
SGOT		58			109			
SGPT								

FIGURE 12-13.   Sean (Case 13)

	3/10/92	6/4/92	7/11/92	8/10/92		
WBC	5.8	5.2	4.9	4.3		
RBC	5.69	5.58	5.3			
HGB	14.4	14.5	13.7	14.6		
HCT	45	44.2	42.4	43.9		
Triglycerides						
Albumin						
Platelets	211	213	208	221		
ESR or sed rate	/	/	/	/		
T4 %	30.5	30	29	29		
T4 #	458	460	551	464		
T8 %	46	53	51	54		
T8 #	691	636	551	854		
CD4/CD8 ratio	.66	.57	.57	.54		
Beta-2 micro-globulin		2.8	2.5	2.8		
P24 antigen						
P24 antibody						
Neopterin						
SGOT		82	27	27		
SGPT		163	47	41		

mended AZT. Sean decided to consult with me before putting together a treatment plan. My recommendations were blue-green algae, lysine owing to a history of herpes, NAC, and a short period on AZT. In just one month, his T_4 cells rose to 551 and the AZT was discontinued. His liver enzymes went all the way down into the normal range, a response I've seen in many people who take blue-green algae. His T_4 cells then decreased to 464 in August 1992, but the percentage did not change and the ratio did not change that drastically. At that point I recommended adding Tagamet and naltrexone, agreeing with the client that going back on AZT at that time was premature.

Case 14: Alice

Alice is a thirty-three-year-old Hispanic substance abuser. She recently entered drug treatment to stop using crack and other drugs. When I met her, in June 1991, her T_4 cells were 341 and I recommended immune modulators—Tagamet, naltrexone, and Antabuse. She was not interested in AZT or other alternative therapies. Her T_4 cells—count, percentage, and ratio—all went up into a very comfortable range (the T_4-cell count above 500).

Case 15: Tom

A thirty-year-old white male, Tom was interested in only natural alternative therapies when I met him in April 1992. I recommended blue-green algae, NAC, lysine, B_{12}, Flora Balance (acidophilus), and two weeks on a garlic regimen. He was complaining of gas and stomach cramps, symptoms that can be a sign of parasites, and one of the best uses for garlic is for parasitic infections. His percentage of T cells went up slightly, as did his ratio. These measurements have continued to rise since July 1992.

Case 16: Jose

Jose came to me in June 1991 with 313 T_4 cells. His doctor had recommended AZT, but Jose did not wish to explore this option at that time. I recommended naltrexone, Antabuse, Tagamet, Zovirax (600 mg daily), and blue-green algae. His T_4 cells immediately rose more than 100 points, and they continued to rise. Currently, they are in the 600 range, and Jose is thinking of

FIGURE 12-14.   Alice (Case 14)

	6/11/91	1/8/92		
WBC	2.80	2.40		
RBC	4.20	3.87		
HGB	12.8	14.0		
HCT	39.1	40.1		
Triglycerides				
Albumin				
Platelets	297.0	285.		
ESR or sed rate				
T4 %	35.0	39		
T4 #	341	542		
T8 %	39.0	37		
T8 #	381	515		
CD4/CD8 ratio	.89	1.05		
Beta-2 micro-globulin	/	/		
P24 antigen	/	/		
P24 antibody	/	/		
Neopterin	/	/		
SGOT	/	/		
SGPT	/	/		

FIGURE 12-15.   Tom (Case 15)

	4/13/92	7/9/92		
WBC	4.2	4.4		
RBC	3.27	4.04		
HGB	12.4	14.8		
HCT	35.3	43.0		
Triglycerides				
Albumin				
Platelets	159	152		
ESR or sed rate	/	10		
T4 %	29	31		
T4 #	341	414		
T8 %	/	/		
T8 #	/	/		
CD4/CD8 ratio	.50	.60		
Beta-2 micro-globulin	1.8	1.8		
P24 antigen	16			
P24 antibody	17,405			
Neopterin				
SGOT	20	19		
SGPT	13	13		

FIGURE 12-16.   Jose (Case 16)

	6/28/91	8/29/91		
WBC	5.8	6.7		
RBC	/	4.74		
HGB	16.0	15.7		
HCT	47.2	44.1		
Triglycerides				
Albumin				
Platelets	241	251		
ESR or sed rate				
T4 %		21		
T4 #	313	468		
T8 %		61		
T8 #		1360		
CD4/CD8 ratio	.35	.34		
Beta-2 micro-globulin				
P24 antigen				
P24 antibody				
Neopterin				
SGOT	19			
SGPT	18			

discontinuing the Tagamet, naltrexone, and Antabuse and staying with only the most natural, nontoxic therapies.

Case 17: Irving

Irving was a forty-four-year-old white male who had 612 T cells and whose doctor recommended no intervention. He came to me because he wanted to maintain his health and impede further progression of the virus. This is probably the best possible time to intervene—you have plenty of time to explore all the natural interventions, your back is not against the wall, and you can keep trying until you find a treatment that works for you. My recommendations to Irving were blue-green algae, vitamin C, and intranasal B_{12}. We saw results immediately—Irving's T4 cells rose more than 100 points.

Case 18: Leo

Leo is a twenty-six-year-old white male. He learned that he was HIV+ in 1990, and he saw his T4 cells decline to 368 by July 1991, when he met me. His doctor had advised him to do nothing; his T4-cell count was considered high and his P24-antibody count was extremely high (his early P24-antibody count was unavailable for this chart). I advised Leo to intervene with a few options no matter what his doctor advised, pointing out to him that it would be easier to maintain his health than to rebuild it following a further decline in his T4 cells.

He did not want to intercede with any toxic substances, so together we decided on a regimen of vitamin C, blue-green algae, and B_{12}. Leo also began taking lysine, because of consistent herpes cold sores in his mouth. After he began the regimen, his T4 cells rose on two labworks and continued to rise. They are now comfortably above 500. Leo is extremely involved in a career that he is devoted to and loves. In addition, the final bloodwork on this chart showed a beta-2 count that had gone down slightly and an antibody count of 3,100, well above the 1,000 mark, which is considered very good.

Case 19: Jacques

Jacques is a thirty-five-year-old European male who came to me when his T4 cells went to 275 after consistent decreases on AZT. I

FIGURE 12-17.   Irving (Case 17)

	2/18/92	5/20/92		
WBC	5.1	7.1		
RBC	4.24	4.04		
HGB	13.6	12.9		
HCT	38.4	36.7		
Triglycerides				
Albumin				
Platelets	205	227		
ESR or sed rate	/	/		
T4 %	30	32		
T4 #	612	727		
T8 %	48	51		
T8 #	914	1159		
CD4/CD8 ratio	.63	.63		
Beta-2 micro-globulin				
P24 antigen				
P24 antibody				
Neopterin				
SGOT				
SGPT				

FIGURE 12-18.   Leo (Case 18)

	7/30/91	11/21/91	4/10/92		
WBC		4.03	4.1		
RBC		5.11	4.63		
HGB		15.7	14.3		
HCT		45.9	42.1		
Triglycerides					
Albumin					
Platelets		181	199		
ESR or sed rate	/	/	14		
T$_4$ %	36	32	32		
T$_4$ #	368	402	471		
T$_8$ %	42	50	52		
T$_8$ #	429	679	765		
CD$_4$/CD$_8$ ratio	.86	.64	.62		
Beta-2 micro-globulin	1.9	2.1	1.9		
P$_24$ antigen			—		
P$_24$ antibody			3100		
Neopterin					
SGOT			40		
SGPT			28		

FIGURE 12-19.   Jacques (Case 19)

	7/1/91	10/21/91	9/11/92		
WBC	4.4	4.2	4.3		
RBC	3.85	3.93	3.46		
HGB	12.0	12.6	10.8		
HCT	35.8	36.2	33.0		
Triglycerides					
Albumin					
Platelets	128	144	117		
ESR or sed rate	38	47	29		
T4 %	16	18	19		
T4 #	275	363	327		
T8 %					
T8 #	1428	1633	1359		
CD4/CD8 ratio	.19	.22	.24		
Beta-2 micro-globulin	/	/	/		
P24 antigen					
P24 antibody					
Neopterin					
SGOT			26		
SGPT					

suggested he try ddI along with blue-green algae and B_{12}. Initially, his T cells went up to 363 and then went down to 327, but even though the T4 cells decreased, the T4-cell percentage went up, and so did the ratio. With these positive results canceling out the drop in T4-cell count, I do not consider this a change for the worse. This is a good illustration of why it is important to look at more than one count before making treatment decisions. After getting these results, Jacques added naltrexone, Antabuse, and Tagamet to his regimen, and his T4 cells, percentage, and ratio all rose, with the T4-cell count going above 400.

Case 20: John

John, a Hispanic male of thirty-five, came to me after he had been on AZT for more than eighteen months. He had started with 500 T4 cells, and by the time of our consultation, he had 258. I recommended that he immediately discontinue the AZT, and he did not want to try any other nucleoside analogue options (ddI or ddC). I recommended lysine, blue-green algae, and Enhance (an herbal formula), and suggested that he might later consider taking gamma globulin, Tagamet, and naltrexone. After he started the regimen, his T4 cells went to 377 and he decided to stick with the same regimen at that time.

Case 21: Elliot

Elliot came to me when he learned he was HIV+. A very high-strung person, he was extremely upset over this news. His agitation and high stress level were evident, and I strongly recommended that he consult a psychotherapist to help him process the news of his HIV status. I recommended blue-green algae and Peptide T. He immediately saw rises in his T4-cell count, percentage, and ratio. In addition, his P24 antibodies were 32,939, which is extremely high, an excellent sign.

FIGURE 12-20.   John (Case 20)

	5/92	7/92		
WBC	6.3	6.9		
RBC	3.22	5.42		
HGB	14.4	15.0		
HCT	41.8	45.5		
Triglycerides				
Albumin				
Platelets	156	268		
ESR or sed rate				
T4 %	9	13		
T4 #	258	377		
T8 %				
T8 #				
CD4/CD8 ratio	.12	.17		
Beta-2 micro-globulin		2.3		
P24 antigen				
P24 antibody				
Neopterin				
SGOT				
SGPT				

FIGURE 12-21. Elliot (Case 21)

	5/92	7/92		
WBC	4.70	4.70		
RBC	4.60			
HGB	14.1			
HCT	41.7			
Triglycerides				
Albumin				
Platelets	546			
ESR or sed rate				
T4 %	24	25		
T4 #	308	400		
T8 %	58			
T8 #	746			
CD4/CD8 ratio	.41	.42		
Beta-2 micro-globulin	/	2.3		
P24 antigen	/	26		
P24 antibody	/	32939		
Neopterin	/	/		
SGOT	/	/		
SGPT	/	/		

SUMMARY

I hope this information has given you a sense of the scope of your options and their possible combinations. Remember, even the greatest medical scientists do not have all the answers regarding the treatment of HIV infection. You need to become your own researcher—and the monitor of your own treatment.

Believing in and feeling comfortable with your treatment options are important cofactors. And tracking your bloodwork is quite possibly the best way to monitor any treatment's efficacy.

CHAPTER 13

OI Treatments

Minor opportunistic infections can begin to occur when T4 cells drop below 500, with the more serious infections occurring below 200. It is rare for OIs to occur when T4 cells are above 500, or even between 250 and 500. Effective drug regimens exist for most of the opportunistic infections, and, as I explained in an earlier chapter, certain drug treatments help protect against development of opportunistic infections. The most common prophylaxis (preventive) treatment is Bactrim, for PCP pneumonia.

Treatments for opportunistic infections are complex and frequently vary with the specific circumstances. In this chapter, I list infections related to HIV and treatment options, but in many cases I omit dosing and drug combinations, since different manifestations and different levels of severity must be treated differently. If you are interested in obtaining specific information on how to treat these infections, see the descriptions of *The AmFAR Directory, The AIDS Knowledge Base,* and *The Medical Management of AIDS* in Chapter 19.

The cause of opportunistic infections is the deterioration and weakening of the immune system. There are various theories on how HIV weakens the immune system and even *if* HIV is the cause for the weakening, but the effect is certain: the immune system is weakened. So the goal in controlling HIV is threefold:

---

* *Note:* Most HIV+ people with T4 cells above 500 have no need for the information in Chapters 13 and 14. Usually, serious OIs do not occur until T4 cells are below 300. I have placed these chapters after the information that all HIV+ people need so that you can skip them and go on to Part III if they do not pertain to you.

TABLE 13-1   Opportunistic Infections

Note: The infections are listed in order of frequency of occurrence, with the most common first. For more information on OIs, see the tables in Chapter 4.

Infection	Treatments
Pneumocystis carinii pneumonia (PCP)	Bactrim, Septra, IV pentamidine, dapsone
Kaposi's sarcoma (KS)	cryotherapy, vinblastine, alpha interferon, radiation, combination therapeutic regimen
toxoplasmosis	pyrimethamine, clindamycin, sulfadiazine
tuberculosis (TB)	isoniazid (INH), ethambutol, pyrazinamide, rifampin, streptomycin

TABLE 13-1   Opportunistic Infections (continued)

Possible Side Effects	Comments
The most common side effects of Bactrim and Septra are skin rashes and upset stomach. Other side effects are headache, fever, diarrhea, nausea, and vomiting. Dapsone can cause nausea and vomiting, low platelet count, and allergies. Pentamidine can cause low blood sugar, decreased blood pressure, pancreatitis, decreased white blood count, and decreased platelet count.	Bactrim, Septra, and dapsone all cause phototoxicity—which is toxicity to the sun—and people taking these drugs should avoid all sun exposure. This doesn't mean you should avoid walking down the street, but any HIV+ person, on these drugs or not, should avoid long periods of tanning. Dapsone absorption can be a problem when the drug is mixed with certain other HIV medications—for example, ddI. Ask your doctor for additional information on this.
For all these treatments: flu-like symptoms, diarrhea, increased urination, vomiting, headache, constipation, hair loss, weight loss, cramps	SP-PG and AGM-1470 are angiogenesis inhibitors that have been tested by Dr. Paul Gallo, a noted HIV researcher, and show miraculous results in the treatment of KS. This treatment is still experimental, but again, pressure on the FDA could get these drugs on the market sooner, or at least available to people who need them on an expanded-access program.
Pyrimethamine—loss of appetite, vomiting, nausea, anemia Sulfadiazine—headache, fever, chills, diarrhea, vomiting, loss of appetite, nausea Clindamycin—diarrhea, abdominal cramps, skin rash, unusual thirst, weakness, tiredness	These drugs are usually given in combination—for example, pyrimethamine and clindamycin or pyrimethamine and sulfadiazine. In studies, folinic acid is added to prevent deficiency. Diarrhea was common on this combination.
INH—fever, swollen glands, peripheral neuropathy (should be given with B$_6$ to prevent deficiency) Ethambutol—headache, dizziness, confusion, joint	Since there is a strain of tuberculosis (MDR-TB) that is multidrug-resistant, these drugs should be given in combination for a long period, usually a year. One regimen was two months of INH, rifampin, and pyrazinamide followed by four to seven months of INH and rifampin. The CDC has advised that HIV+ people receive at least nine to twelve months of

TABLE 13-1　Opportunistic Infections (continued)

Infection	Treatments
tuberculosis (continued)	
MAI (*Mycobacterium avium* intracellular) or MAC (*Mycobacterium avium* complex)—both names refer to the same syndrome	azithromycin, clarithromycin, ciprofloxacin, clofazimine, amikacin, Rifabutin, rifampin, ethambutol
cytomegalovirus (CMV)	Foscovir (foscarnet), ganciclovir (DHPG)

TABLE 13-1 Opportunistic Infections (continued)

Possible Side Effects	*Comments*
pain, anemia, rash, nausea, vomiting, abdominal pain, fever Pyrazinamide—liver injury and gout Rifampin—liver damage and stomach upset Streptomycin—hearing loss, decreased potassium, impaired kidney function	combination therapy. Check sputum regularly for cultures; if negative three times it is usually safe to go on a maintenance, as opposed to a treatment, regimen. Check with your health-care provider before going on a maintenance regimen.
Can include stomach upset, diarrhea, and rashes	These drugs are usually well tolerated. Up to 1992, we did not have an effective treatment for MAC and people would often become very seriously ill from this infection. Since the approval of clarithromycin and azithromycin, this condition has become manageable, and these treatments work wonderfully. Often, drugs are given in combination—for example, clarithromycin and ciprofloxacin for the first two to three weeks, followed by a maintenance dose of clarithromycin indefinitely.
Foscarnet—kidney damage, problems with mineral levels in the blood, lowered blood-cell count, nausea, tingling in the extremities, tiredness, headache Ganciclovir—lowered white blood count, lowered platelets, bone-marrow depression, elevated liver enzymes, nausea, edema, muscle aches, headache, disorientation, rash, phlebitis	Both of these drugs are difficult to work with and must be administered intravenously. Often, a catheter, which is a central line into a vein, is installed in the chest for administering these treatments. In this case, it is *very important* that the person keep the catheter clean to avoid infection. According to studies, foscarnet recipients seem to live longer and do better, but ganciclovir (DHPG) seems less difficult to administer and has fewer side effects. I suggest that you try to avoid CMV at all costs by doing aggressive CMV prophylaxis early on, including high-dose acyclovir. There is a lot of controversy over whether or not that prophylaxis works, but the bottom line is that people live longer on acyclovir. I would even suggest you consider weekly IV of ganciclovir, which a small study has shown to be an effective prophylaxis for CMV. Check your CMV titers (through a blood test by the same name), and if they are rising and your T4 cells are below 100, this is a reasonable option. But note: DHPG cannot be taken with AZT, since both drugs cause bone-marrow depression. See Chapter 14 for information on prophylaxis.

TABLE 13-1   Opportunistic Infections (continued)

Infection	Treatments
cryptococcal infection (meningitis)	amphotericin B, fluconazole
candidiasis, candida, thrush	clotrimazole, fluconazole (Diflucan), itraconazole, ketoconazole, nystatin
herpes simplex/herpes zoster (shingles)	acyclovir (Zovirax)
wasting syndrome	Megace, Marinol, total parenteral nutrition (TPN), Trental
HIV encephalopathy (dementia)	AZT, Peptide T

TABLE 13-1   Opportunistic Infections (continued)

Possible Side Effects	*Comments*
Amphotericin B—fever, chills, nausea, anorexia, pain at infusion site, anemia, kidney problems Fluconazole—stomach upset, rash, headache	Amphotericin B is given intravenously for this infection and is extremely invasive, often causing chills, fevers, and shakes. Fluconazole is tolerated much better, but physicians are reluctant to use it first, because it is slightly less effective and may take longer to work. If this infection is caught early on, fluconazole can be used much more effectively. One study at the AIDS conference in Amsterdam (PoB 3186) cited 800 mg daily of fluconazole as an effective treatment for cryptococcal meningitis. This study initiated treatment with a 1,600-mg daily loading dose. Prophylaxis with fluconazole can be extremely effective (see Chapter 14).
The side effects may vary from drug to drug, but all the treatments share these side effects: diarrhea, stomach pain, nausea.	Side effects to these treatments are minimal and the drugs are extremely effective in treating candidiasis infections.
Skin rash, diarrhea, lightheadedness, headache, nausea, vomiting, thirst, fatigue	Although side effects are listed, they do not seem to be common among users of this drug. High doses—3,200 to 4,000 mg daily—are definitely recommended for people with fewer than 100 T4 cells, or fewer than 150 if there is a history of herpes and CMV titer is rising.
Dizziness, disorientation, one reported fever; side effects are rare. New studies with Trental have doubled the original dose from 400 mg three times a day to 800 mg three times a day. This high dose can cause eye problems. All drugs should be discussed with your health-care professional.	Megace and Marinol are appetite stimulants. TPN is an intravenous drip of high-caloric nutrients. Trental works on restoring proper absorption of food.
AZT—bone-marrow suppression, headaches, abdominal pain Peptide T—the growth of extra hair and heightened libido	This is one of the best uses for AZT. Unfortunately, the drug is usually given long before symptoms of dementia arise, rendering it ineffective by the time it is needed. Peptide T, available only through buyers clubs, remains the most effective and least toxic treatment for HIV-related encephalopathy (dementia).

TABLE 13-1   Opportunistic Infections (continued)

Infection	Treatments
cryptosporidiosis	diclazuril, azithromycin, somatostatin, paromomycin (Humatin)
hairy leukoplakia	acyclovir (Zovirax)
syphilis	penicillin
human papillomavirus (HPV; anogenital neoplasms)	carbon dioxide laser, cryotherapy, electrocautery, excision and surgery, radiation treatment, systemic chemotherapy
peripheral neuropathy	Elavil, mexiletine, Peptide T
lymphoma	Treatments vary depending on type of lymphoma.
histoplasmosis	amphotericin B, ketoconazole, itraconazole

TABLE 13-1 Opportunistic Infections (continued)

Possible Side Effects	*Comments*
Little or no toxicity is reported with these drugs. Some of them are still experimental, so little information is available.	*Paromomycin*, according to the *AmFAR Treatment Directory*, seems to be the most effective treatment for this condition. Unfortunately, this drug is not yet available. Out of these drugs, paromomycin (brand name Humatin) and diclazuril are available through an expanded-access program from the drug company. Azithromycin is available by prescription.
skin rash, diarrhea, light-headedness, nausea, vomiting, thirst, fatigue	Most doctors will say that there is no treatment for this condition, but according to the AmFAR directory, investigators have noted that oral high-dose acylovir, 3 grams daily, can reduce or eliminate hairy leukoplakia lesions. Usually, patients begin with 800 mg of acyclovir, adding 800 mg every week until the hairy leukoplakia lesions begin to disappear. It can happen at lower doses as well.
Minimal	Latent syphilis is a problem in HIV infection. If syphilis recurs, aggressive IV therapy is recommended by the CDC; I agree with their recommendation.
Toxicity differs depending on treatment. Often painful at the site where the drug is administered.	Treatment may also include local chemotherapy with cytotoxic agents, which burn off the warts.
Elavil: tiredness Mexiletine: heart problems	Because mexiletine and Elavil both have side effects and are effective in relieving treatment in only about 50 percent of users, Peptide T remains the treatment of preference. Peptide T has been studied in people with peripheral neuropathy with good results, and this drug is also readily available through buyers clubs. For trials, call 1-800-TRIALS-A.
Chemotherapeutic and radiation treatments have side effects such as nausea, vomiting, weight loss, and hair loss.	Most HIV-related lymphomas are extremely treatable and are easily put into remission.
Amphotericin B is usually associated with chills, shakes, fevers, and other flu-type symptoms. The other drugs have fewer side effects.	No treatment has been found to be completely effective against histoplasmosis, but amphotericin B has been shown effective in controlling the clinical manifestations.

1. treating infections (the major part of the effort)
2. rebuilding the immune system
3. stopping the virus

If you are dealing with opportunistic infections and attempting to develop a treatment regimen, be aware that a well-rounded treatment program must include an antiviral and immune modulator as well as specific OI treatments.

The table beginning on page 246 covers four types of information:

- the name of the infection
- the treatments currently available
- possible toxicities
- comments

You need to explore any toxicities with your doctor, because the toxicities listed on the table occur in only a small number of cases. Therefore, accurate information is important. If your doctor gives you fear-inducing information about treatment options—or about HIV infection in general—you might do yourself and other patients a favor by pointing out to the doctor the effect of what he or she is saying, and explaining how your fear could undermine both your efforts to stop the progression of the virus and your positive attitude.

The infections I list in Table 13-1 are HIV-related and AIDS-related. To determine whether an infection is AIDS-related or HIV-related, refer to Tables 4-1 and 4-4 in Chapter 4.

For people whose T4 cells are above 250, most of the information on this table will be irrelevant, but you might want to familiarize yourself with it anyway or look up specific infections.

SUMMARY

Most opportunistic infections are treatable. In the spectrum of HIV infection, HIV+ people seem to be most vulnerable to OIs when T4 cells fall below 100. Many HIV+ people can prolong the period when T4 cells are above 100.

If the information you are seeking is not in this chapter, you should be able to find it in the resources listed in Chapter 19. Remember, immune modulation and antiviral therapy are extremely important in preventing recurrence, no matter what opportunistic infection you are dealing with.

CHAPTER 14

Preventive Therapy

Prophylaxis is, quite simply, preventive therapy. It means that you take a drug to prevent the development of an infection—in this case, quite serious opportunistic infections. Although prophylaxis therapy is merely prevention and should be practiced by anyone in any health situation, it is still a new idea in Western medicine.

If you are HIV+ and your T cells are under 200, the information in this chapter on infection-preventing therapies is crucial. If your T cells are above 500 to 700, then following the recommendations in the natural-therapies chapters might prevent you from ever reaching the point where you need the information in this chapter. So, in essence,

- prevention early in HIV infection means preventing further proliferation of the virus, minimizing your susceptibility to infection, and halting deterioration of your immune system;
- prevention later on means taking measures specifically designed to inhibit the development of specific opportunistic infections.

* *Note:* The table in this chapter not only outlines prophylaxis therapies for advanced HIV infection, but also offers overall treatment recommendations for HIV infections broken down by T4-cell categories.

With this distinction clear in your mind, you can see that many therapies may be preventive. For example, acupuncture early on in HIV infection can help people stabilize and maintain their health. In China, acupuncture is used for health maintenance, and therefore prevents people from getting sick—an approach that still remains foreign to the philosophy and practice of Western medicine. If we were to begin using, for example, vitamins, acupuncture, and blue-green algae to keep us healthy and to prevent disease, we could very possibly ease the stress on the health-care system and alleviate our current insurance and medical-management problems. But at this point—as is the case in all arenas, not just the medical one—Western ideas of problem-solving are oriented strictly toward crisis intervention, not toward the larger picture and long-term results.

As you know by now, in the course of HIV infection, if the immune system is compromised opportunistic diseases or infections can occur. These opportunistic infections are quite serious and sometimes difficult to treat. Therefore, the medical management of HIV infection includes therapies to prevent acute active manifestations of some OIs. I say "some" because only some regimens have been proven effective; others are still being tested; and for some OIs (for example, PML [see Table 4-4]) no prophylaxis treatments are being tested at all.

Two distinct approaches to prevention fall into the category of prophylaxis:

- *Primary prophylaxis* are drugs or supplements given when T4 cells or other blood tests indicate a rise in susceptibility to an opportunistic infection.
- *Secondary prophylaxis* are drugs given to patients who had a particular OI infection to prevent its recurrence.

But, although the distinction seems fairly straightforward, the practice of prophylaxis can be extremely complicated. People with compromised immune systems might be taking ten to twenty medications plus supplements—a situation that itself, in my view, severely limits the quality of life. So I encourage people who are trying to decide whether or not to add a prophylaxis therapy to read widely, collect all the relevant information, and arrive at a decision carefully with respect to the total treatment picture. Prevention has been proven to work and can dramatically limit the number of opportunistic infections a person might have in the course of HIV infection.

Just looking at T4 cells is not a sufficient criterion for deciding whether or not to incorporate some of the prophylaxis interventions in your treatment regimen. However, most of the recommendations are indicated by T4-cell counts alone. In this chapter, I try to broaden the recommendations by including other blood tests and symptomology.

It has been my experience that some doctors, when prescribing prophylaxis, forget about the central problem, which is twofold:

- stopping the virus
- rebuilding the immune system

Frequently, in consultations, I see patients who are at a particular recommendation borderline—i.e., their T4 cells are at 240, which could be a time for prophylaxis against PCP, while above 250 no prophylaxis is recommended. In these borderline cases, I often recommend aggressive immune modulation and antiviral therapy plus increased medical monitoring—up to once every three weeks—to rebuild the immune system, increasing the patient's T4 counts well out of the realm where the prophylaxis is recommended. So, instead of adding the PCP prophylaxis, we use more-aggressive monitoring, antiviral treatments, and immune-modulating drugs to bring the client's T4 cells over the borderline and out of the level at which prophylaxis is recommended. In this way we sidestep the need for the additional medication. To repeat: Many practitioners who prescribe prophylaxis therapy forget that while you are taking drugs to prevent diseases, you also need to be on

- antiviral therapy to stop the virus
- and an immune-modulating therapy to rebuild the immune system.

As your own advocate and informed participant in your medical-treatment program, you are in the position to make sure you are receiving treatment and attention on every front.

PROPHYLAXIS THERAPIES

To simplify the recommendations for prophylaxis, I have organized them into a table. Also for the purpose of simplification, I
have used the T_4-cell count as the basic criterion, including other
indicators where possible. Remember, the decision-making
around prophylaxis is neither simple nor cut-and-dried, so I
strongly recommend that you not only consult your health-care
professional but that you do additional reading as well.

A study reported at the Eighth International AIDS Conference
indicated that combinations of prophylaxis therapies were effective and that side effects resulting from drug interactions did not
seem to be a problem (PoB 3144). The drugs tested were Bactrim
or dapsone for PCP prophylaxis, pyrimethamine for toxoplasmosis prophylaxis, fluconazole for fungus, acyclovir for
herpes and possibly CMV, and clarithromycin with ciprofloxacin
for MAI or MAC. Of the 88 patients tested, 28 patients experienced 36 adverse effects and no one in the study developed any
of the opportunistic infections they were prophylaxed against.
All participants had fewer than 250 T_4 cells, average T_4 count
was 48, 47 subjects had prior OIs, and the mean time on the
regimen was 8.8 months. The table contains the recommendations from this study as well as other recommendations.

But before presenting the particulars of these treatments, two
pieces of information deserve mention that don't fit into Table
14-1:

1) If your T_4 cells are above 500 and you have a history of
herpes infections, or if your T cells are between 500 and 800 and
you had chickenpox when you were a child, I recommend 1,500
mg daily of lysine, an amino acid, as a possible prophylaxis
against herpes and herpes zoster (shingles). There is no documentation that lysine can prevent herpes zoster (shingles), but
there is information that lysine reduces the number of herpes
attacks and their severity in people with herpes who take

- 1,500 mg daily in three doses—that is, 500 mg 3 times daily.

In addition, there is some evidence that herpes is a definite
cofactor in the activation of the HIV virus—that is, with active

herpes present, HIV proliferates at an increased rate. With this additional information, and with lysine being a nontoxic amino-acid supplement, this therapy seems to make sense. This treatment would follow the historic development of prophylaxis recommendations, which are usually low doses of the drugs used for treatment of the infection.

Acyclovir, or Zovirax (a brand name), is the other therapy used to prevent herpes, and there is more documentation of its efficacy than there is for lysine. But for people with T cells above 500, acyclovir, a nucleoside analogue, seems much too aggressive.

2) The other recommendation not covered on the table is for people, and especially women, with a history of vaginal yeast infections, or yeast infections in the mouth (thrush). Again we see candida, which causes these infections, as a cofactor in the proliferation of HIV, straining the immune system and therefore minimizing its effectiveness against HIV. Prophylaxing against these yeast infections in a natural way can help eliminate this underlying infection. For people with more than 500 T cells, acidophilus, a natural substance discussed in Chapter 8, is used to prevent recurrent yeast infections and in some cases is taken just to keep the body balanced, to correct digestion, and to prevent diarrhea. If you currently have a yeast infection, you should first treat it with the recommended medications listed in Chapter 13 (Table 13-1) and then consider the natural therapies discussed in Chapter 8 to prevent additional yeast infections.

SUMMARY

Certainly prophylaxes can be difficult and extremely complicated, and the amount of drugs that people sometimes wind up taking definitely minimizes the quality of life. To help you sort through this complex information, I recommend that you concentrate on three major prophylaxes:

- PCP prophylaxis
- MAC prophylaxis
- CMV prophylaxis

with the other prophylaxis regimens added as needed.

Again, to design an effective regimen of prevention, you

should discuss the treatments with your doctor and collect all information about them as it emerges.

TABLE 14-1   Prophylactic Therapies

For T4 Cells Between 300 and 500

- Have regular bloodwork done every three months.
- Have PPD skin tests for TB along with an anergy panel (see Chapter 5). Often, the PPD is nonreactive owing to a compromised immune system; the anergy panel verifies the PPD results by measuring immune-system capability. Also, PPD response should measure 5 mm to be considered positive (measured by a small ruler-like instrument), but since weakened immune response is common in HIV infection, many doctors consider any response to be a positive response. If anergy panel is negative, the first action is to rule out active TB by chest X ray, exam, and a careful medical history. If PPD is positive but there are no symptoms of active TB, standard prophylaxis against tuberculosis would be
    —300 mg of isoniazid (INH) daily, with 50 mg daily of vitamin B_6 (also known as pyridoxine) for one year
- Regular vaginal exams every six months to test for candidiasis, and Pap smear. Colposcopy should be included at least once a year to compensate for Pap smear irregularity. Any history of current vaginal yeast should be treated with
    —clotrimazole cream or fluconazole once daily for two weeks, or
    —Mycelex vaginal suppositories
    To prevent recurrence, add
    —acidophilus three times a day (some HIV OB-GYN specialists recommend inserting the acidophilus vaginally, one tablet per week; check with your health-care specialist)
    If recurrent herpes is a problem, and 1,500 mg of lysine daily is not effective,
    —200 mg of acyclovir three times daily is recommended, and has been found to be more effective than 200 mg two times daily (PoB 3331).
- Consider Pneumovax inoculation for pneumonia if not previously inoculated. Bacterial pneumonias are common in HIV infection; in fact, recurring bacterial pneumonia is one of the categories the CDC added to its AIDS definition in January 1993.
- Some practitioners recommend a flu shot once a year. Whether this is necessary has engendered a lot of controversy. If you have received one flu shot, you should continue with the yearly vaccination. If your T4 cells are above 600, you might want to do additional research on vaccines before considering a flu shot.
- Consider a vaccination against hepatitis B. HIV+ people are often hepatitis B positive, and this can be a cofactor in the proliferation of HIV infection. If you are hepatitis B negative, a hepatitis B vaccination is recommended.

T4 Cells Between 200 and 300

- If you have any history of herpes, prophylaxis is
    —200 mg of acyclovir three times daily.
Lysine is not recommended with this T4-cell count.

TABLE 14-1   Prophylactic Therapies (continued)

• PCP (*Pneumocystis carinii* pneumonia) prophylaxis is recommended if T cells go below 250 or below 20 percent. This recommendation can be confusing. If your T4 cells are between 300 and 250 and your T4-cell percentage is below 20, then PCP prophylaxis is recommended, but if your T4 cells are between 300 and 200 and your T4-cell percentage is way above 20, then the need for prophylaxis is less likely unless your T4-cell count reaches 225. With T4 cells between 250 and 200, some HIV+s whose percentage is above 22 consider holding off on prophylaxis. Standard prophylaxis for PCP is
—Bactrim DS (double strength) three times weekly,
and that is my recommendation, considering that people on this prophylaxis have the fewest number of new PCP cases reported as compared with other PCP prophylactic treatments. If you are allergic to Bactrim, a Bactrim-desensitizing program can be used with your physician's supervision. The programs usually use a pediatric form of Bactrim liquid, beginning at very low doses and gradually building up dosages over a one-month period.
The second choice for PCP prophylaxis is
—100 mg of dapsone daily.
The third choice is
—aerosolized pentamidine once a month.
Aerosolized pentamidine has a 10–20 percent breakthrough of new cases of PCP. That is why Bactrim and dapsone should be considered before pentamidine.
• When T4-cell count is below 250 or 20 percent, check toxo titer, which measures *Toxoplasma gondii* (the organism that causes toxoplasmosis) activity if you are positive. This test is called a toxo IgG or IgM test. If you are toxo negative, avoid undercooked meat, gardening, and cat feces. (See Chapter 16 for more details.) If your T4 count is below 250, test toxo titer quarterly to see if there is a rise. If the antibody titer begins to rise, most practitioners recommend beginning the standard prophylaxis for toxo, which is
—25–50 mg of pyrimethamine daily, or
—1 double-strength tablet of Bactrim once or twice a day.
There is no conclusive evidence on either prophylaxis; therefore, these recommendations are conservative. *PI Perspective* suggests 25 mg of pyrimethamine 3 times a week. In Europe, Fansidar is also used for toxo and PCP prophylaxis. At the Amsterdam AIDS conference, one study showed
—1 tablet of Fansidar weekly
to be an effective prophylaxis against PCP and toxoplasmosis (PoB 3303). Prophylaxis for toxo is most commonly given when T4 cells drop below 200 and toxo titers, if positive, start rising. If your toxo test is negative, test every six months to make sure no new exposure has caused infection.

T4 Cells Between 100 and 200

• For persistent fungal infections, such as vaginal or oral thrush, skin fungus, or athlete's foot, one study at the 1992 Amsterdam AIDS conference showed
—100 mg of fluconazole biweekly
to be an effective prophylaxis (PoB 3252). Initially, this treatment, which was given daily or three times weekly, was considered dangerous, since it was thought that fungus could become resistant to it, but another study at the conference showed that fluconazole resistance was rare (PoB 3246). If bi-

TABLE 14-1   Prophylactic Therapies (continued)

weekly prophylaxis does not completely prevent the fungus, increase the dose until you reach a point where prophylaxis is effective. First treat the infection with daily fluconazole; then decrease in this manner, making sure the fungus does not recur:

—three times weekly if no recurrence; then
—two times weekly if no recurrence; then
—one time weekly if no recurrence; then
—one time biweekly.

• CMV prophylaxis, not yet definitive, is usually given when T_4 cells fall below 100, or 6 percent, but since a study in Britain showed that high-dosage acyclovir increased survival rates by 50 percent, I usually recommend

—3,200 mg of acyclovir a day, for CMV prophylaxis.

In addition, a CMV titer could be drawn from the blood when T cells are at approximately 200, and if the titer is drawn regularly and increases in the titer are seen, prophylaxis could be started earlier or later, depending on the titer results.

T_4 Cells Below 100

• For people with any history of fungus infections and T cells below 100,
—50–100 mg of fluconazole daily
or, according to a study reported at the 1992 Amsterdam conference,
—200 mg of ketaconazole daily
can be an effective prophylaxis for cryptococcal meningitis (PoB 3261). This prophylaxis might also be effective against histoplasmosis for T_4 cells below 100 or 10 percent.

• When T_4 cells fall below 50, or 5 percent—and I usually play it safe by recommending this prophylaxis when T_4 cells are at 70—according to a 1992 study published by CRIA (Community Research Initiative on AIDS),
—150 mg of Rifabutin daily
is an effective prophylaxis against MAI or MAC. This illness often goes undiagnosed for long periods, causing underlying deterioration of the immune system. In addition, it is very common and therefore important to address with a prophylaxis regimen.

• If you are on
—3,200 mg of acyclovir daily
and CMV titer continues to rise and T_4 cells fall below 50, you should know about a small study in which patients were given
—250 mg of DHPG (ganciclovir) IV daily for those weighing 120 pounds or less, and 500 mg IV daily for those weighing 120 pounds or more; these dosages were administered (daily) for two weeks followed by once-a-week infusions.

Of the 17 people in the study—9 were on ganciclovir and 8 were on placebo—no one developed CMV on this drug, while 4 out of 8 people on placebo developed CMV retinitis within the same period. CMV is extremely difficult to treat and often goes undetected until it has reached crisis proportions; it should be avoided at all costs. CMV and MAI are two underlying HIV infections that cause undetected debilitation for long periods of time. Prophylaxis against these two OIs is essential.

TABLE 14-1   **Prophylactic Therapies (continued)**

• If T_4 cells are below 50 and below 5 percent, 250 mg of Humatin twice daily has been used as prophylactic treatment against cryptosporidiosis. Physicians report success with this prophylaxis, but no documented evidence as to efficacy has yet emerged.

PART III

LIVING WITH HIV INFECTION

CHAPTER 15

Nutrition and HIV

It's not easy to make generalizations about nutrition and HIV. For one thing, people at different stages of HIV infection have different dietary needs. For another, nutritional philosophies differ depending on the nutritionist you talk with. One fairly safe prescription for good nutrition is to eat foods each day that give you the vitamins, minerals, and other things you need to keep your body strong. Unfortunately, the foods available today make it difficult to follow this prescription.

The nutrients and trace minerals in our food originate in the earth's topsoil, but over the last twenty years the topsoil in this country has been depleted of much of its nutritional value. As I mentioned earlier, the nutritionist Lark Lands, Ph.D., suggests that HIV+ people require five times the normal daily minimum requirement of nutrients. Eating organic foods, which are grown under optimum conditions, can give you more nutritional value than supermarket fare, but buying the necessary amount of food in health-food stores is too costly for most people.

Since nutritional deficiencies can induce HIV progression, high doses of a good supplement such as blue-green algae are essential. Blue-green algae is a food source of vitamins, amino acids, trace minerals, and more. It is a naturally balanced, easily absorbed nutritional supplement that, as you know by now, I recommend highly. Most vitamin supplements are made from chemical sources, which are difficult for the body to absorb. A food-source supplement, such as blue-green algae, probably provides nutrients much more effectively because it is absorbed more efficiently.

I don't pretend to be an expert on nutrition, but I have read enough and practiced long enough in the field of HIV infection to be able to provide recommendations and guidelines. In addition, I have asked Laura Landon, a registered dietitian who works with AIDS patients in New York's Bellevue Hospital, to supplement this chapter with a section on nutrition and HIV infection. Note, however, that her wonderfully rich contribution is directed primarily to the needs of people with progressed HIV infection and AIDS, not asymptomatic HIV+s.

BASIC RECOMMENDATIONS

Many different diets are designed to promote healing. One well-known plan followed by many people dealing with illness is macrobiotics. This diet has had a history of success in healing cancerous conditions, but for people with HIV it is deficient in a number of ways:

• Macrobiotics emphasizes low cholesterol intake, but HIV attacks cholesterol, so substantial cholesterol intake is important for HIV+s.
• Macrobiotic food plans dictate low-grade protein, but the immune system consists of cells made from proteins, and concentrated protein foods such as meats provide the best source for maintaining these building blocks.
• Macrobiotics minimizes vitamin B_{12} content, but HIV depletes B_{12}, so a diet high in B_{12}—the best source of which is red meat—is recommended. Also, as you will see, Laura Landon recommends integrating other high-protein foods, such as fish, yogurt, fortified soy milk, and dairy foods, to ensure high protein intake and to meet your nutritional needs.

The principles that govern the macrobiotic diet can be adapted to meet your needs in the context of HIV infection. Essentially, the principles of macrobiotics are these:

• whole grains or grain products make up 50 percent of the total volume of food consumed each day
• vegetables make up 25 percent of the total

- beans make up 15 percent
- seaweed, miso, and assorted condiments make up 10 percent

If you add meat and other proteins to this diet, it becomes a healthful, well-rounded, balanced meal plan for the HIV-asymptomatic person. The idea is to eat a red-meat protein source in small portions—maybe 10 percent of your meal—approximately three times a week.

According to Dr. Alan Pressman, a New York chiropractor and nutritionist, lamb is the recommended meat choice, owing to its high cholesterol and nutritional content. Usually, a high cholesterol level is undesirable, but since the HIV virus tends to deplete the body's cholesterol intake, this recommendation seems sound and many practitioners have adopted it. Many recommend that meat make up 25 percent of the total intake for HIV+s.

Meat provides vitamin B_{12}, which is depleted in many HIV+ people. Not only macrobiotics, but vegetarian diets are often deficient in vitamin B_{12}. If you decide not to eat meat, you'll need to get B_{12} injections or intranasal supplementation (see Chapter 8).

THINGS TO AVOID

If your T4 cells are above 500 and rising, you may not need to follow the recommendations in this chapter. As I hope I've made clear by now, I firmly believe that if something is working, there's no need to fix it. I'd recommend that you adapt the principles outlined above as you see fit; they will result in a balanced, healthful meal plan. Then acquaint yourself with the information that follows on maintaining the body's optimum healing state.

If you have wasting syndrome, which is defined as the loss of 10 percent or more of your body weight within a month for no apparent cause, you should eat any food that is high in calories and that you like or can develop a taste for.

The goal is to maintain optimum nutritional health. To do that, try to avoid the following or, in some cases, consume in moderation:

- *Fast foods and restaurant foods*. Chemicals and other undesirable additives often abound in these foods, thus hindering optimum nutritional gains.

• *Sugars and sweeteners.* People with thrush should be aware that sugar helps thrush grow. Also, artificial sweeteners contain chemicals with unknown side effects, some of which have been identified as carcinogenic. Many nutritionists believe that these products help viruses grow as well. Yet all agree that if wasting syndrome persists, sugar-fortified products, which are high in calories, may be necessary for weight gain.

• *Raw fish, rare red meat, and raw eggs.* These foods can all transmit parasites, toxoplasmosis, and salmonella. In addition, raw fish carries parasites that can cause incessant diarrhea even in the healthiest people. All HIV+s should avoid these raw and rare products. Cooking these foods eliminates the parasites.

• *White flour.* Whole-grain products and products made from whole-grain flour are more nourishing and easier to digest than products made with processed white flour.

• *Preservatives and chemicals.* These additives interfere with the digestive process, reside in the body, and retard bodily responses.

• *Dairy products.* Most nutritionists agree that dairy products are even harder to digest than meat. Dairy products lodge in the intestines and cause mucus to clog the villi—the tiny structures that absorb nutrients from food. Do not overeat foods from this category.

• *Pork and lunch meat.* Most people know that pork is hard to digest and loaded with bacteria that die when cooked but still remain in the product. Furthermore, "lunch meat" is an unknown combination of leftovers and by-products.

• *Raw vegetables and fruits.* For people with fewer than 300 T4 cells, it's important to peel all fruit and steam all vegetables to avoid exposure to the infectious bacteria that reside on raw and nonpeeled foods.

In addition, note the following:

• *Psyllium husk cleansing.* This product, available at any health-food store, is recommended for cleansing the bowel—but only for people with no history of diarrhea. Follow directions on the container. Use the product once in the morning and once in the evening for two weeks every six months. Psyllium husks will not cause a loose movement but will cleanse the bowel, resulting in extended, fuller movements.

• *Protein Supplementation.* Since protein is vital to cell growth, protein supplements are useful and harmless. Most health-food stores carry protein shakes, though many have chemicals and additives you can do without. I recommend the protein shake available through the blue-green algae company my office supplies information on (see Resource Guide). It is vegetarian, without any preservatives or sugar.

• *Water.* Nutritionists recommend that you drink two quarts of water daily—preferably water that has been charcoal-filtered. People with fewer than 100 T4 cells are susceptible to MAI and cryptosporidiosis and should drink carbon-block-filtered or distilled water *only*. I usually recommend these precautions when T4 cells are lower than 300. This is a conservative approach, one that prevents consistent exposure and immune responses to these organisms. The real danger from these bacteria comes when T4 cells are below 100.

TOTAL PARENTERAL NUTRITION (TPN)

Total parenteral nutrition (TPN) is an intravenous feeding method that is an excellent intervention for people with wasting syndrome. Many practitioners wait until the patient is severely debilitated to administer TPN, but this option is better used early on. Project Inform's article on TPN (*P.I. Perspective,* October 1991) recommends this therapy for early intervention to rebuild the body so it can maintain its resistance against germs.

Recent findings reported at the Eighth International AIDS Conference (PoB 3695) showed that albumin loss (the measurement of protein in the blood; see Chapter 5) and usual body-weight loss are predictive of "risk of death" (kind of final, but that's how the conclusions in the study were worded). Subsequently, Donald Kotler, M.D., and nutritionist Lark Lands both connected disease progression to weight loss and nutritional deficiencies.

These developments have stimulated a new line of thinking for me: instead of connecting weight loss to progression, I associate body weight with survival. That weight loss contributes to HIV progression, if not ultimately death itself, seems to be significantly documented. So keeping your weight up becomes a priority, and this small section on TPN takes on new importance. TPN can give you a significant weight increase when you are unable to keep eating enough to keep your weight up on your own. If you are underweight, I urge you to discuss this therapy with your doctor. Try to secure treatment *early,* before active opportunistic infections occur. TPN is an important nontoxic treatment for weight loss that might otherwise contribute substantially to HIV progression.

HOW HIV INHIBITS FOOD ABSORPTION

At a recent HIV nutritional seminar, Donald Kotler, M.D., of St. Luke's Hospital put forth some very interesting theories. These theories, based on his own research, make good sense to me.

First, a little background: In the body, as HIV infection progresses, TNF (tumor necrosis factor) levels rise and glutathione levels drop. These two factors seem to inhibit the proper absorption of food and, possibly, the absorption of medication used to overcome HIV infection. In Chapters 8 and 10, I described two interventions—NAC and Trental—that seem to restore TNF and glutathione levels to normal.

Another measurement—of albumin, a protein in the blood (discussed in Chapter 5)—is used to track the progression of wasting syndrome. A decline in albumin level means a loss of protein in the blood, and this is considered a sign of wasting syndrome. A decline in albumin level has also been linked to the progression of HIV infection (PoB 3695). It is with the link between nutritional wasting and HIV progression that Dr. Kotler concerned himself in his recent lecture.

After reviewing reports of people who died of starvation, Dr. Kotler found that death occurred at the point where the person declined to between 60 and 66 percent of his or her normal body weight. Noting that many HIV+ people live for an indeterminate period with a wide range of opportunistic infections, he also found that people with AIDS (PWAs) who reached 60 to 66 percent of their usual body weight died more readily. His findings suggest a strong link between death from HIV infection and usual body weight. Dr. Kotler cautiously pointed out that his results were preliminary and needed more study, but the theory was certainly worth considering.

After considering these theories, I began to follow weight and albumin levels in my HIV clients. This in turn has led me to use TPN earlier and more aggressively than is usually the case to prevent further weight loss. Appetite-stimulating drugs are help-ful for the same reason, and Trental and NAC can be used aggressively to reverse some of the conditions that may inhibit the absorption of nutrients.

APPETITE-STIMULATING DRUGS

Two drugs are used to stimulate the appetite of people who are having trouble maintaining their weight. Both these drugs seem to work well, and people do gain weight on them. Still, these drug treatments deal more with the symptoms of wasting syndrome—poor appetite—rather than with the cause, which is poor food absorption.

• *Megace (megestrol acetate)*. This drug is used to treat advanced breast cancer in women. It changes the hormonal balance of the body, and in doing so causes constant feelings of hunger. In one study published in the *Annals of Internal Medicine* all patients on Megace gained weight at an average of 1.1 pounds per week. The dosage is 300 to 600 mg/daily.

According to Dr. Kotler, Megace does have possible drawbacks. He explained that Megace can lower the testosterone level, a little-known fact. Many people with weight loss from HIV infec-tion already have a lowered testosterone level, a depletion that itself can interfere with the absorption of food. So even though Megace is effective in treating the symptoms of wasting syn-drome, it may well exacerbate the very cause of the weight loss. Dr. Kotler recommended that testosterone levels be measured and tracked in patients with wasting syndrome and suggested that these patients might even receive testosterone supplementa-tion when the level is below normal. But when asked if this meant he would reduce the number of Megace prescriptions he writes, Dr. Kotler responded with an emphatic no.

• *Marinol (dronabinol)*. This drug contains the active ingredient in marijuana, which also stimulates appetite. It has been used as an antinausea treatment for cancer patients on chemotherapy. The most effective dose cited by the drug company marketing Marinol is

• 2.5 mg twice daily.

Some patients experience lethargy or tiredness on Marinol similar to the effects of marijuana.

I have gathered these general recommendations over ten years of research, observation, reading, and clinical experience. The following section, by Laura Landon, covers the specific recommendations most mainstream dietitians currently use for patients in the later stages of HIV infection, usually people with AIDS. If you are asymptomatic, the information that follows may not apply to you, and you should follow the recommendations in the first half of the chapter. But let me end with a cautionary note: There are as many diets as there are nutritionists in the United States. Approach them all, and especially the vegetarian diets, with care. Remember that HIV can deplete the protein, vitamin B_{12}, and cholesterol you need as an HIV+ person. Make sure you discuss your nutritional intake with a nutritional counselor you can trust.

NUTRITIONAL INTERVENTIONS WITH PROGRESSED HIV INFECTION

Laura Landon is a registered dietitian who works as an AIDS nutrition specialist in New York's Bellevue Hospital. She wrote this material, which continues through the end of the chapter, for PWAs and HIV-symptomatic people who have experienced a decline in body weight.

Nutrition affects immunity, so it is crucial that HIV+s at all stages of infection learn about and practice good nutrition, and nutrition customized to their particular needs. In particular, deficiencies of protein, calories, vitamins, and minerals can interfere with immune function.

Inadequate intake of the first two factors—protein and calories—can result in a condition called protein/calorie malnutrition (PCM). PCM occurs when unplanned weight loss is severe and body-protein stores deplete. Following Nick's advice in monitoring your labwork can help you prevent or turn PCM around. The lab result indicating the level of stored body protein is the serum albumin reading. A measurement of less than 3.0 gdl indicates protein depletion of the visceral organs such as the heart, liver, lungs, and kidneys as well as the skeletal muscles.

If you remember that muscles are made up of protein, you'll understand why it is imperative to monitor the serum albumin level and respond nutritionally when the readings go down. When protein and calories are insufficient to build and repair muscle, the size of muscles diminishes.

Before the HIV pandemic, PCM was one of the most common causes of immune-system weakening. In 1987, the Centers for Disease Control classified HIV infection with wasting syndrome (a weight loss of 10 percent or more over a one-month period) as a diagnosis of AIDS.

PCM comes about in HIV infection for a number of reasons:

- fever
- infections
- diminished food intake owing to difficulty or pain in chewing and/or swallowing, loss of appetite, nausea, vomiting, and diarrhea

More than one of these causes can be present simultaneously.

The role of nutrition for HIV+ people is to prevent weight loss so that the immune system stays healthy. If you are HIV+ and asymptomatic, the best thing you can do is eat a well-balanced diet that is high in calories and protein. Table 15-1 lists the minimum recommended servings for PWAs or adults with HIV-related weight loss and gives examples of foods in the four basic food groups.

Although eating a balanced diet can help provide adequate protein, vitamins, and minerals, you may need to increase calories to prevent weight loss.

If you begin to lose weight, here are some suggestions:*

- If your food intake is not maintaining your weight, you are probably not getting enough vitamins and minerals. I recommend one to two "one-a-day" type supplements that contain approximately 50 to 150 percent of the recommended daily allowance (RDA) for vitamins and minerals.
- Eat at least three meals a day plus snacks. Use the "basic four food groups" in Table 15-1 as a guide.

TABLE 15-1   **Minimum Recommended Servings for PWAs or Adults with HIV-Related Weight Loss***

Food Group	No. Servings a Day	Rich in	Sources
1. Milk	2 or more	Protein, calcium, riboflavin	Milk, cheese, pudding, ice cream, yogurt
2. Meat	2 or more	Protein, niacin, iron, thiamine	Meat, poultry, fish, eggs, or substitute cheese, beans, peanut butter
3. Fruit and vegetables	4	Vitamins A & C	Raw, cooked, or juices of; citrus fruits and dark green, leafy veggies
4. Grain	4 or more	Carbohydrate, iron, thiamine, niacin	Breads, cereals, pasta, rice, potatoes

* Adapted with permission from D. Rakower, "Nutrition and HIV," in *Bellevue Hospital Center AIDS Patient Handbook,* J. Kalinoski, ed. (New York: New York City Health and Hospitals Corporation, 1991).

• Eat calorie- and protein-dense foods and snacks—for example:
  • cheese and crackers
  • hard-boiled eggs
  • dips and chips
  • ice cream and toppings
  • peanut butter and crackers
  • fruited yogurt

• Eat double the usual amount of meat on a sandwich.
• Add cheese to sandwiches as well as meat.
• Eat protein foods first (see Table 15-1); it will be easier to digest and be assimilated more effectively that way. This food will not only have the most protein, but if it's fried, it will have the most calories, too.
• Add fat and sugar to foods to gain extra calories. For example, add butter and/or cheese, cream, and gravies to potatoes, rice, noodles, and vegetables; also, use extra sugar and heavy cream in coffee and milk shakes.
• To keep from filling up on fluid instead of food, save drinks for the end of meals. HIV+ people often feel full before the end of a meal. To prevent early satiety from reducing your food

intake, eat many small meals throughout the day rather than several large ones.

- Supplement your meals with:
—puddings
—milk shakes
—liquid supplements such as Sustacal, Resource Plus, Ensure Plus, and Nutrament; taking in these supplements between meals can help maintain weight

- Add powdered milk or instant-breakfast powder to whole milk and milk products.
- Avoid low-calorie foods and beverages—such as tea, coffee, broth, and lettuce salads—that might fill you up.

NUTRITIONAL RESPONSES TO OIS

If you are dealing with opportunistic infections, you may want to consult with a registered dietitian (RD) for an assessment of the nutritional issues associated with your condition. The RD will assess disturbances in food intake, absorption, and metabolism that can result in protein-calorie malnutrition and then counsel you in how to respond with specific nutritional interventions.

The most common nutritional problems associated with a diminished food intake are difficult or painful chewing and/or swallowing. Oral and esophageal candidiasis, Kaposi's sarcoma, cytomegalovirus (CMV), and oral herpes simplex all interfere with food consumption. Table 15-2 offers suggestions for responding to this and the other food-consumption problems associated with HIV infection.

TABLE 15-2 **Solutions to Eating Problems***

Loss of appetite. Precede meals with relaxation techniques. Take small, frequent, calorie- and protein-dense meals. You might want to ask your doctor for an appetite stimulant such as Megace.

Nausea. Choose cold, bland, dry foods. Also try such cold foods as tuna or chicken salad, cottage cheese, and fruit. Eat and drink slowly. Ask your doctor to prescribe an antinausea medication; take this as needed a half hour before meals. Eat toast, crackers, pretzels, or cookies. Avoid greasy, spicy, or strong-smelling foods.

TABLE 15-2   Solutions to Eating Problems (continued)

Vomiting. During episodes of vomiting, avoid solid foods and maintain a liquid diet of clear liquids (broth, apple juice, Jell-O, tea with sugar, ginger ale, Popsicles, and ice). Eat when vomiting has subsided. Rest after eating, but don't lie flat. Drink clear liquids between meals. As with nausea, ask your doctor for an antinausea medication. If certain medications bother your stomach, take them with food or antacids.

Diarrhea. Drink plenty of liquids between meals to replace lost fluid. Gatorade can help replace fluids and minerals. For sudden-onset diarrhea, try bananas, rice, applesauce, and tea temporarily. For ongoing diarrhea, avoid high-fiber, gassy, greasy, fried, and fatty foods. Dairy foods may be causing diarrhea; ask your doctor or dietitian about lactose-intolerance and lactose-free products. For severe ongoing diarrhea, total parenteral nutrition (TPN) may be medically appropriate.

Early satiety (a feeling of the stomach filling quickly). Avoid liquids before meals and eat small, frequent meals.

Difficulty swallowing. Take soft, blenderized, pureed, or prepared baby foods as tolerated along with calorie- and protein-dense supplements. Prepare soft foods such as mashed potatoes, egg omelets with cheese, custards, cooked cereal, yogurt, cottage cheese, flaked fish, ground meat, casseroles, tuna or egg salad, and milk shakes. Moisten food with butter, gravy, and cream sauces. Use a cup instead of a spoon when eating soup and cereal. Avoid very hot foods.

Painful swallowing. Same as above, but avoid foods that cause pain (for example: soda bubbles; spicy, salty, and rough foods; raw vegetables and fruits, especially citrus fruits; sticky, dry food such as peanut butter).

Difficult or painful chewing. Same as for *Difficulty swallowing*, above. Ask your doctor about prescribing a viscous lidocaine (to numb the affected area) you can swish in your mouth before meals.

Taste changes. Add flavors to foods by mixing in (with vegetables) ham strips, bacon bits, chopped onions, or cheese sauce. Try such herbs as basil, oregano, rosemary, tarragon, and mint. Serve food cold or at room temperature.

Shortness of breath. Use a nasal cannula—a tube that delivers oxygen—during meals if medically appropriate.

Dementia. Secure help with meals.

Strict dietary restrictions. Consult a registered dietitian, who will be able to assess individual needs and customize a menu plan.

Inadequate funds for foods. Ask a social worker for help. You may be eligible for public assistance such as Medicaid and food stamps. Many communities have free meal programs.

Too tired to prepare food. Keep snack foods handy. Prepare simple meals such as

TABLE 15-2   Solutions to Eating Problems (continued)

meat and cheese sandwiches, hamburgers, sliced meat heated and served with gravy, scrambled eggs with cheese, and tuna salad. Use convenience foods such as TV dinners, pizza, fish sticks, canned soups, beef stew, and fruits and vegetables. If you can afford it, buy take-out food.

DEALING WITH DIARRHEA

More than 50 percent of symptomatic HIV+ people have diarrhea, a condition that can result in severe weight loss owing to the malabsorption of food. There are many causes of HIV-related diarrhea and, to respond effectively, it is important to determine the cause of the diarrhea and whether it involves malabsorption.

Organisms in the system are a common cause of diarrhea. Possible organisms include:

- *Cryptosporidium*
- *Isopsora belli*
- microsporidia
- *Giardia lamblia*
- CMV

Kaposi's sarcoma in the gastrointestinal tract can result in malabsorption.

Another cause of diarrhea is gastrointestinal infection. Such an infection is likely to limit nutrient intake, which can result in protein caloric malnutrition. When infections and malnutrition occur, it is virtually impossible for the person to get enough calories, and a downward cycle of weight loss can result. In such a case it may be necessary to use a nasogastric tube—a tube placed in the nose—to deliver nutrients directly to the stomach or duodenum.

Food poisoning is another possible cause of diarrhea. You can decrease your risk of food-borne infections by following these suggestions:*

- Avoid rare meat; medium- and well-done meats involve less risk of contamination.

* Adapted with permission from D. Rakower, "Nutrition and HIV," in *Bellevue Hospital Center AIDS Patient Handbook*, J. Kalinoski, ed. (New York: New York City Health and Hospitals Corporation, 1991).

- Avoid store-bought meat, chicken, and tuna salads made with mayonnaise. These spoil easily.
- Avoid raw eggs (for example, in unpasteurized eggnog, Caesar salad, the drink "poche," and so on). Raw eggs can carry salmonella. Cook your eggs for at least four minutes to kill the germs. Well-done eggs are safest.
- Refrigerate leftovers quickly.
- Reheat foods thoroughly.
- When in doubt, if food looks or smells spoiled, throw it out.
- Avoid raw, unpasteurized milk or milk products.
- Do not use "organic" lettuce, since fertilizers used with these products contain infectious organisms that remain on the lettuce.

THE IMPORTANCE OF TPN

When a person is not ingesting or absorbing a sufficient number of calories, total parenteral nutrition, described earlier in this chapter, becomes a possible option. I personally recommend TPN when a person's nutritional needs are greater than the amount of nutrients that can be delivered by mouth or through a nasogastric tube. Usually, the need to use TPN results from:

- gastrointestinal disorders such as chronic intestinal cryptosporidiosis or microsporidiosis
- severe esophageal ulcers
- malabsorption of carbohydrates and fat

TPN can retard weight loss in people with systemic illness such as MAI/MAC or CMV infection where weight declines despite aggressive nutritional support. Nick describes early intervention with TPN, which up until now has been used in tertiary stages. Using TPN early on *can* prevent or delay nutritional deficiencies resulting in protein caloric malnutrition. This practice is becoming more widely available as information on the relationship between weight loss and HIV progression increases.

CHAPTER 16

Infection Control

What does *infection control* mean to you? This chapter doesn't have anything to do with the spread of HIV infection. We have already established how HIV is transmitted and prevented. Rather, this chapter is geared toward avoiding exposure to infections—what are called *opportunistic infections* in the context of a weakened immune system. You can avoid developing many of the serious opportunistic infections associated with HIV by avoiding exposure to them. For example, just by practicing safer sex and using a condom, you can avoid exposure not only to HIV but also to many sexually transmitted diseases (STDs), CMV, herpes, HPV (human papillomavirus), and others.

As you can see, the practice of safer sex protects against more than just the transmission of HIV. Theories about Kaposi's sarcoma, or KS, suggest that it too might be spread sexually or through oral-anal contact. So safer sex, if it becomes the norm, will prevent the spread not only of HIV, but of many of the opportunistic infections associated with HIV.

In a similar vein, in learning how particular infections are transmitted, we have come up with specific prevention practices. Here's a survey of the measures to take to prevent particular OIs:

• *CMV (cytomegalovirus)* is spread through mucous-membrane contact, sexual contact, and tissue or blood transfusions. Practice safer-sex measures and avoid direct contact with infected tissues or blood.

• *Cryptococcosis* is a yeastlike fungus found worldwide, often in soil that is contaminated with bird excrement. Simply wearing gloves and a mask while digging in the garden prevents exposure to this infection.

• *Cryptosporidiosis* is spread through fecal/oral contact. The causative agent is a parasite that can contaminate food or water everywhere, so it's necessary to boil all water and cook all food.

• *Histoplasmosis* is transmitted through inhalation of soil particles contaminated by bird droppings or other organic material. Ninety percent of HIV+ people diagnosed with histoplasmosis have T_4 cells below 100.

• *MAI (mycobacterium avium intracellulare)* or *MAC (mycobacterium avium complex)* is found in soil, food, and water. Simply cooking food and boiling water prevents exposure to these germs.

• *TB (tuberculosis)* is on the rise in the HIV-infected community and is spread by breathing in infectious particles. Good ventilation in all rooms, especially with someone who is actively coughing, decreases the possibility of exposure to the airborne respiratory secretions that spread tuberculosis. Have a PPD, a TB skin test, regularly. (See Chapter 5.)

• *Toxoplasmosis* can be spread through raw or undercooked meat, especially lamb or pork. Wash your hands after handling raw meat or vegetables and wear gloves while working in the garden.

Also, change cat litter daily. Cat feces becomes infectious for toxoplasmosis forty-eight hours after it is dropped, so if you change the litter daily—and as an extra precaution wear gloves and a protective mask while doing so—you can avoid breathing in or taking in the causative agent of toxoplasmosis.

For the same reason, avoid pigeon feces as well.

GENERAL INFECTION-CONTROL PROCEDURES

Most people who become infected with the above conditions have T_4 cells below 100, so if your T cells are dropping, it's absolutely essential that you take the precautions described. But there are certain infection-control procedures that everyone should follow, regardless of bloodwork results. These practices are bound to sound familiar—they're just the sorts of things your parents probably drummed into your head when you were young. But in the effort to protect yourself against opportunistic infections associated with HIV, it can be useful to reacquaint yourself with these general principles of infection control:

• *Wash your hands.* Most infections are spread when the hands pick up an infectious agent that is then inhaled or put into contact with a mucous membrane (often the eyes). Simply avoiding contact and washing your hands regularly can minimize the transmission of many infections, including the common cold. When washing your hands, rub them for at least twenty seconds; the friction is the main germ-eliminator in this practice.

• *Keep properly hydrated.* In plain English, drink enough water, at least two quarts a day. Water helps your primary defense, your skin, stay properly moisturized and free of little cuts or other openings where infections can enter.

• *Use a moisturizer* for the same reason you should drink enough water. Common, over-the-counter skin moisturizers help close little cuts in dry skin through which infectious agents can enter the body.

• *Don't share utensils or cigarettes.* I hope that most of you have stopped smoking by now, but this rule is just common sense. Many infectious conditions, such as the common cold and tuberculosis, can be spread this way.

• *Make sure you have adequate air circulation in your room.* It is a good idea to have an effective window fan in your room that pulls fresh air in through the window or pushes stale air out of the room. Constantly changing the air in the room reduces your risk of inhaling airborne infections.

• *Avoid cat feces, bird droppings, and the water in fish tanks.* No matter what your T4-cell count, let somebody else do the actual cleaning up around your pets. All these substances carry infectious agents.

• *Do not handle soil—or, if you must, wear gloves and a mask.* Again, no matter what your T4-cell level, avoiding exposure to the infectious materials in soil can prevent problems down the line. In addition, each exposure to a germ would cause an immune response, which would have the potential to activate HIV residing in the immune system.

• *Take precautions in interactions with infected people.* Many of us know people who are HIV+ and visit them often. Taking the proper precautions in no way means you should minimize your contact with people. The human touch can have its own healing powers, for both the giver and the receiver. Also, taking *unnecessary* precautions, such as wearing protective masks, gloves, and gowns in the presence of infected people, can be downright detrimental by conveying negativity, pessimism, and fear. But you can still reduce the spread of infection by washing your hands after touching a person who is actively ill or making sure there's proper ventilation in the room. Opening the windows or doors in a stuffy room will not only reduce your chances of picking up an infection, it could do the sick person a lot of good also.

Some people might have infections—for example, shingles (herpes zoster)—that produce sores on the body. The general rule about sores is that if they are open and oozing, they are probably contagious, and this is certainly true of shingles. The use of rubber gloves for contact is absolutely necessary and can prevent the transfer of infectious agents.

• *Use a disinfectant.* Disinfectant kills invisible organisms.

• *Do not share towels or personal-care items.* Use one towel a day. Proper towel use will prevent the spread of common fungal infections on the skin.

• *Clean toothbrushes with peroxide and water once a week.* Soaking your toothbrush once a week for fifteen minutes in a solution of one-quarter peroxide to three-quarters water will kill any infectious material that might have collected on it.

Using common sense to avoid infections is an important part of stopping HIV progression. As we go about in the world, we are all exposed to infectious agents in air, water, and food, and exposure to these agents triggers immune responses within our bodies. Each time your immune system mounts a response, its strength for fighting HIV is diluted. In addition, HIV lives within the immune system; activating the system (when your body responds to infection) can potentially activate HIV replication. Avoiding daily exposure to parasites and inhaled agents of infections as much as possible and keeping your immune system strong are positive control measures you can take to inhibit the progression of HIV.

CHAPTER 17

The Mind–Body Connection: Psychoneuroimmunology

We are each 100 percent responsible for all of our experiences.

—Louise L. Hay
You Can Heal Your Life

When we think of healing we usually think of physical healing, but "A Course in Miracles" defines health as inner peace. There are people experiencing critical illness who are at peace, and people in perfect physical health who are emotionally tortured.

—Marianne Williamson
A Return to Love

THE FOUR QUESTIONS

At first a patient's emotions and attitudes might not be fully accessible to consciousness. To retrieve them, I found that we need to explore the answers to four basic questions.

1. Do you want to live to be a hundred?
2. What happened to you in the year or two before your illness?
3. What does the illness mean to you?

4. Why did you need the illness?
>   —BERNIE S. SIEGEL, M.D.
>   *Love, Medicine, and Miracles*

The AIDS patients who live long past the time predicted for them seem to have certain traits in common. Perhaps the most important of these characteristics is the refusal to accept the verdict of a grim inevitability. . . . They do not accept the fatalism so characteristic in public thinking about the disease. They provide emotional support for one another. Their personal horizons are uncluttered by defeatism and inevitability.

>   —NORMAN COUSINS
>   *Head First: The Biology of Hope*

With love for ourselves and for each other, we shall heal this planet of fear and dis-ease. When this experience is over, every person on this planet will have been touched, and many will have been changed in a positive way. It is time for us to all live and practice unconditional love. Love will enable the world to take a quantum leap into a new and magnificent future.

>   —LOUISE L. HAY
>   *AIDS: Creating a Positive Approach*

There is no death. The son of God is free.
>   —*A Course in Miracles*

For years scientists have speculated on the possibility that by sharply focusing our attention we could use our minds to control and in many situations heal the body. Scientists such as Bernie Siegel have tracked people who have had experiences of such self-healing. Louise Hay has actually cured herself of cancer. Many, many people have written books and papers attesting to their self-healing powers, and some simply walk around silently knowing that in some way they have participated in their healing much more fully than by simply taking a pill.

My work with HIV+ people and this book are rooted in my certainty that the mind plays an important role, a role that must not be underestimated, in the body's healing. For Louise Hay, illness is a message from our bodies telling us that something in our reality is wrong—perhaps we need to forgive someone, to clear up some past pain, or just start learning how to love ourselves and others. I say *just* need to love ourselves, but I don't use that word to minimize the importance of loving ourselves. Loving ourselves and holding on to that love are major tasks, the greatest challenges we face.

It is both exciting and encouraging that theories that have circulated for centuries regarding the mind–body connection are now being scientifically proven by a new science. This field, called *psychoneuroimmunology,* actually studies how the mind can influence the body's healing process. Even more exciting, and specific to HIV infection, is the finding in Dr. Mary Anne Fletcher's University of Miami study (mentioned earlier) that a routine of exercise, meditation, and stress reduction increased immune function and immune cells, including T_4 cells. As a matter of fact, this routine resulted in an increase as great as that brought about by AZT over the same amount of time. And this was not a small study. It was a major study with a control group— as explained before, a group on a placebo that is compared with the group using the routine being studied. In this case, one group of approximately 200 people did an exercise/meditation/stress-reduction routine and one group did not. The group that did the routine had significant increases in immune action and T-cell production. Fletcher was so excited by the findings that she asked that her grants be extended so she could continue her research. The National Institute of Mental Health denied the grants.

As a society—a capitalistic one, I should add—we have turned our backs on the potential healing benefits that

- are free
- are accessible
- take inner work to achieve

When you design your holistic treatment plan—which addresses and draws from mind, body, and spirit—if you do not identify and work on the issues of your life that make you unhappy, stress you out, or cause you to feel as if you want to die, you are overlooking a significant factor in your healing process.

In September 1988, the New York *Daily News* went out on a limb and printed an article in its magazine section called "Why Do Some People Survive AIDS?" This article followed several people who had been diagnosed three years or more before with ARC or AIDS and were alive and "in remission." In June 1990, the *Daily News* went back to visit those same people. Out of sixteen people covered earlier, thirteen of the people were still alive. Three were experiencing some health problems, but most were asymptomatic.

What accounted for these encouraging survival stories? In Michael Callen's *Surviving AIDS,* the author also tracked survivors—the people he covered had survived an AIDS diagnosis for three years or more. Callen isolated seven characteristics shared by all the survivors he tracked:

1. Survivors are realistic about the seriousness of their condition without being fatalistic. They refuse to believe AIDS is an "automatic death sentence."
2. Survivors are willing to take responsibility for their own healing and to make major life-style adjustments to "accommodate disease in an adaptive way." Survivors believe that physical fitness and exercise contribute to healing and further believe that their "personalized means of active coping" can have "beneficial health effects."
3. Survivors tend to have extraordinary relationships with their health-care providers. They spoke of a healing partnership with their health-care providers, and were neither passively compliant nor defiant.
4. Survivors are passionately committed to living and have a sense of "meaningfulness and purpose in life," of "unmet goals." Often, the diagnosis itself enables them to find "new meaning" to life.
5. Survivors tend to have faced and overcome past life crises.
6. Survivors deemed it important to meet and talk, especially shortly after their own diagnosis, with other people with AIDS in a supportive environment. They also considered it beneficial to be "altruistically involved" with other people with AIDS—being self-concerned without being exclusively self-involved.
7. Survivors are assertive and able to communicate openly, which includes having the ability to say no. Survivors "nurture" themselves and are "sensitive to their body and its needs."

SO HOW DOES IT ALL WORK?

Although there is more and more evidence that our immune system is affected by our emotions, the science of how precisely the emotional aspects of our being communicate with our immune system is new and sketchy. This science, psychoneuroimmunology, begins by focusing on the brain, the controller of the human body. Most of the brain's communication work is conducted through neurons. These cells are too small to be measured or weighed. Estimates of the number of neurons in the brain are constantly changing. Current estimates range between 40 and 50 billion.

The neurons carry traffic for millions of signals. Some three dozen secretions are produced or activated by the brain through these neurons. The brain also has the ability to combine these secretions in thousands of combinations. Certain secretions, such as endorphins and enkephalins, which act as the body's own painkillers, may also regulate immune function. Another secretion, interferon, can trigger immunological functions and combat infection.

Candace Pert, Ph.D., formerly of the National Institute of Mental Health, has identified neuropeptides as substances through which the brain and body intercommunicate. Dr. Pert has described emotions as stimulating the release of neuropeptides that either support or hinder the immune response. For example, stress and worry produce neuropeptides that hinder immune response, while self-love and happiness produce neuropeptides that support it. A case in point is endorphin, the neuropeptide released during aerobic exercise. This peptide functions not only as the body's painkiller but also to enhance and stimulate the function of killer cells within the immune system. Neuropeptides are probably responsible for the effects of emotions on the immune system.

Stress reduction, visualization, and certain other techniques stimulate a type of body–mind communication that increases the activity of a wide range of immune cells. Incorporating these techniques into your treatment plan to combat HIV infection can only help add to the benefits you experience from that plan. Many books are available that describe these techniques, and I have included a section on them in the Resource Guide. The bulk of this chapter will cover some basic self-healing principles that are widely incorporated and have proven effective in the treatment of illness.

PSYCHOTHERAPY

Much of the existing self-healing material suggests that unexpressed or unresolved emotional conflicts may contribute to the proliferation of illness. For instance, Louise Hay links the abuse she experienced as a child to her development of cancer later in life. She saw cancer as resentment growing within her in the form of a tumor. This link between past emotional trauma and illness is not uncommon, and therefore the self-healing community and its literature advocates the developing of a therapeutic relationship with a professional psychotherapist.

A Course in Miracles, which is a self-study psychotherapeutic spiritual path, also addresses psychotherapy in its literature. It implies that psychotherapy and spirituality are connected by a common goal: to make the mind work perfectly. So, in a spiritual setting, if your mind is working perfectly, then you are in touch with the God within. Likewise, in psychotherapy, if your mind is working perfectly, your life runs more smoothly.

Psychotherapy helps the mind work properly by freeing up buried feelings through communication. Anxiety, overwhelming feelings of fear, despair, and other forms of emotional distress dissipate when they are shared. When I am overcome by negative emotions, I turn to a list of people who form my support network. Often, I go down the list until someone says something to me that strikes a chord and begins to make me feel better. The things you hold inside and don't communicate can become stressors that subsequently create negative physical conditions. What are ulcers? They are feelings and emotions that are not communicated and remain bottled up inside.

Talking is only one form of communication, but there are many ways of dealing with distressing emotions. Some people write, some paint, some meditate, some go into a room and scream. Some people count to ten, some people eat, and others might take drugs. I'm not suggesting you should take drugs or drink to release your emotions, but there will be occasions when you'll need to let off steam. If you respond to an impasse by having a few drinks before waking up the next morning and dealing directly with the problem, I don't consider that extremely unhealthy, emotionally. Physically, though, for the HIV+ person, a couple of drinks can create an environment in which HIV replicates more readily.

On a very real level, strong negative emotion can deprive you of the ability to think straight. When we become angry or fearful, we experience a physiological reaction called the fight-or-flight response. This response sends extra blood to our hands and feet, reducing blood flow to the brain. Did you ever get so angry you couldn't think? All you could do was scream and yell? Often, when you see people fighting, what do they say? They curse, they say things that are hurtful. In these circumstances, they aren't really thinking, since the brain cannot think when it is deprived of blood and oxygen. Instead, they are able to express only old, negative responses. When you feel angry and are in the fight-or-flight response, counting to ten and breathing deeply allows the oxygen to reenter the brain so you can begin to think clearly. Even sucking a lollipop would do it—anything that gives you the time to bring blood and oxygen back into your brain.

But even once the thoughts have been cleared, communicating anger is difficult. We need to learn to say what's on our minds in a reasonable tone *while* we are angry. This takes practice. Also, underneath the anger there may be a multitude of other feelings that need to be expressed. You're often hurt when you're angry, and it is the expression of *this* emotion that will give you a sense of relief and resolution if you can manage to reach it.

Psychotherapists are wonderful for helping people deal with anger and other distressing emotional states. Remember, a problem shared is half a problem. And a joy shared is twice the amount of joy. While acupuncture, chiropractic, massage, and exercise all have a place in your healing regimen, psychotherapy in one form or another might well contribute to your body's ability to fight infection.

In working with HIV+ people, I suggest a range of psychotherapeutic strategies:

- talking to a good friend
- participating in a good support group
- using a professional psychotherapist

The most important criterion for choosing a group or a person in whom you can confide your emotions is a positive outlook on HIV infection. You need to be able to rest assured that doom and gloom and negativity are not the basis for the group and that the person will not undermine your confidence in your efforts to heal yourself.

Using this criterion doesn't mean that anyone who mentions death or dying is negative. It is not negative to acknowledge death and dying as possibilities. But if you pick up a hint or suggestion that the person or group you are considering sees death as the *only* possible outcome of HIV infection, quickly reject that route and look elsewhere.

Most HIV+ people's attitudes toward HIV infection fall into one of two categories, and you can usually get a sense of where people are at just from hearing a sentence or two. I call these two distinct categories the "Ifs" and the "Whens." People in the first group say, "*If* I get sick, I'll look into selling my life insurance for profit." This group leaves the possibilities open—they might get sick; then again, they might not. The second group says, "*When* I get sick, I'll look into selling my . . ." This group recognizes only one possible ending—illness and probable death. Which group are you in?

Your local community-based HIV organizations can probably give you referrals to groups or psychotherapists who deal with HIV infection in a positive way. If you are lucky enough to be near New York or Los Angeles, a group called the Healing Circle, started by Louise Hay in Los Angeles and a group of her followers in New York, is one of the best contexts in which to practice self-healing techniques. The Healing Circle focuses on healing from within, on the premise that if the mind is healed the body follows. Remember, the focus of this approach is spiritual, emotional, and mental healing, *not* the healing of the body. Though many techniques are available, all rest on a single premise: Heal the mind and the body might follow. But even if it doesn't, the practice itself helps you become so wonderfully tuned in to life that you will find a way to accept whatever happens to you. This acceptance reduces stress and fear while allowing a quality of life few people ever get to experience.

DEATH AND DYING

Many PWAs get sick so many times that their "will to live" deteriorates and they gradually begin to accept death. Others see death from the beginning as the only possible outcome to their infection, and still others see death as a possibility but not the *only* possibility. No matter where your own attitudes fall in this spectrum, accepting your own mortality and confronting the loss of HIV+ friends and loved ones are unavoidable issues.

Twelve-step programs state that "fear is a lack of faith." Living with a life-threatening illness can produce levels of fear unknown to you until then, but fostering spiritual beliefs can help you live with that fear one day at a time. Consciously cultivating spiritual strength can help you put into perspective the fear of death or the fear of the form death might take. On the strength of their beliefs, many HIV+s have found comfort by beginning to look at death as a part of life, as a door to another phase of life.

Our society is usually in denial of mortality. Most people are completely out of touch with death as a possibility for them, even though they have experienced the deaths of others. Unlike most HIV+ people who have had their denial shattered by finding out they are HIV+, all of us can use help in acknowledging that death is a part of life, and therapy is a great resource for this.

Acknowledging the possibility of death and living a day at a time, without dwelling on negativity, can help you cope with fear. In self-healing, you are usually encouraged to maintain a positive thought—but this need not mean that you deny the possibilities . . . *all* the possibilities.

It's worth adding here that the comforting value of spiritual beliefs does not begin and end with the fear of death. Spiritual awareness and faith enhance the quality of life in general and add depth to relationships, sometimes heightening life experiences to near perfection.

AFFIRMATIONS

We are constantly talking to ourselves in our own minds. Many of the things we say to ourselves tend to scare us, worry us, and create fear in our lives. An affirmation is any statement you make to yourself that can ultimately end up determining emotional states. When you think a thought, the thought stimulates a kind of discussion in your mind, and the discussion brings about an emotion. This series of events might happen so quickly that you might not even notice it, and some of the sentences you repeat to yourself might be so inbred, having been learned and reinforced over many years, that you don't even have to say them consciously—they just repeat automatically. All such statements are affirmations.

Taking negative statements, turning them around, and repeating positive statements to yourself tends to reduce the stress in your life and foster a positive attitude that can enrich your quality of life. Many metaphysical teachers go beyond claiming that affirmations merely reduce stress to assert that affirmations can create a reality. For example, "I am sick, I am sick" can create the reality of being sick. "I have no money, I'm not worth it" creates the realities of no job and no money. Whether affirmations really create the states described or reduce stress only minimally, they are definitely a positive addition to anyone's life.

If you walk around all day saying, "I have AIDS; I'm going to die," don't you think you're going to feel stressed? But, if you walk around saying, "I am alive, I am healthy, I am safe," you can reduce your level of stress and quite possibly create a more positive physical reality.

George Melton, who wrote *Beyond AIDS* (Brotherhood Press, 1988) with Will Garcia, used these techniques to create a remission from symptomatic HIV infection. After Melton was diagnosed, he immediately began trying every remedy that appeared to have an effect against HIV. Since AZT had not yet been approved, the choice of medical intervention was not just limited, it was nonexistent. He flew to Mexico for Ribavirum and Isoprinsine, which later showed no benefit after testing. He then began to search for answers within.

His efforts amounted to an all-out spiritual search. He read anything he could get his hands on, from Edgar Cayce to Louise Hay. He began working with the principles of affirmation and visualization, and not only did his symptoms begin to disappear, but his life started to take on a new meaning. He began to travel the country, sharing his experiences through lectures, and in the course of his travels he discovered a new way to live—built on giving and receiving love. Currently, George Melton lives in California, where he continues to thrive.

With respect to technique, it's important to cast affirmations into the present tense. It's not "I *will* be healthy"; it's "I *am* healthy." Statements about the future tend to remain in the future. If your intention is to create health and prosperity for yourself, you need to do that in the *now*.

I've used affirmations in my life many times. The first step is to lie back and look at my thoughts—and when I do this I often find negative statements about myself. In the past, when these thoughts floated through, I tended to believe them: "I'm not going to get the job. I don't have a degree." But when I went to a workshop with Louise Hay, she shared the fact that she had been a high-school dropout and had never gone to college. For a long time, she told us, she had believed that that would hold her back—and it did.

When she told this story, I realized she was talking about me. I *really* heard what she was saying—and at that point I decided that the fact that I had not graduated from college would not hold me back any longer. Within six months, after doing a lot of inner work and creating affirmations for myself, I tripled my salary. Some time later, I got my degree but for my own personal enrichment, not to get a better job.

The following principle applies in any area of life: To make changes, you need to be aware of the problems. If you rush through life and never take a moment to understand and be aware of what exactly your head is saying to you, you will not have the ability to change it.

My mind was saying to me, "I'm not a college graduate. I won't get the job." I changed those thoughts, using these affirmations:

- "I am intelligent just the way I am."
- "I'm a wonderful person with a lot to give."
- "I love myself."
- "My income is constantly increasing."

In the area of health, here are some sample affirmations to try:

- "I am healthy."
- "I am safe."
- As Bernie Siegel would say, "All hands that touch me are healing hands."

- "I am capable of making positive medical decisions."
- "I bless all my medications."
- "These medications are making me well."
- "My T4 cells are constantly increasing."
- "I am abundantly healthy."
- "I am strong and healthy."

MEDITATION

Edgar Cayce said that ten minutes of meditation a day can change your life. The workbook for *A Course in Miracles* is composed of 365 daily meditations that train you to release a thought system of fear and adopt a thought system of love. In my own life, if I meditate for fifteen minutes a day, I am more centered, things don't upset me as easily, I am able to communicate my feelings more easily, and I feel generally less stressed than if I simply go on my way without taking the time for myself.

There are many different ways to meditate. Louise Hay once defined meditation as "creating the space to listen to your own internal wisdom." Inside each one of us are many different voices, but if we remain quiet we can hear a voice that is deep down at our core, and that voice is what many people call God. Others refer to it as an Inner Guide, a Higher Self—call it what you will. A great many people rely on that voice in making their health-care decisions. I personally appreciate the benefits of clearing my mind, reminding myself that I am safe, and centering myself through daily meditation.

Some people do visualizations during their meditations. In this technique, you picture what you want to be true. So, if you wish to create perfect health, during a quiet meditative state you picture yourself in perfect health. Or you might picture yourself getting better, or picture your body mounting a response to the virus, or—one of my favorites—picture the thymus gland, which is in the throat, producing many, many new T4 cells. Each person searches and comes to his or her own visualizations. Many tapes and books are available and many techniques have been developed to help you customize your visualizations to your specific needs.

George Melton, long-term survivor, speaks of finding his way through the ocean of techniques and advice and choosing those he thought he could follow by selecting only those that rang true for him on a gut level. Each of us has a definite instinct for recognizing what's best for us, but to uncover that instinct takes daily practice and emotional support.

Did you ever have a really bad feeling and then experience something awful? Eight days before my father died, I had a premonition that he was going to die. This is a common experience that originates in a part of ourselves that most of us are not generally in touch with. During the healing process, many people get in touch with a deep internal guidance, which helps them toward health. Many spiritual paths teach that God wants for you only perfect health, perfect happiness, and a wonderful life. You need only open yourself to those intentions.

CHAPTER 18

On the Horizon

For many years I was extremely hopeful that a cure for HIV infection would surface in the research and be approved quickly. But now it seems that researchers have let the search for a cure drop out of their sights. I don't mean to inject a negative tone here, because there are certainly many options for HIV+ people to follow up on, but I do want to draw attention to our current limitations.

Most current research is designed to seek treatments for HIV infection or for HIV-related diseases, *not a cure*. Treatment will certainly be welcomed, making HIV a manageable chronic illness much like diabetes—although I propose that for those with the proper information this is the case right now. But it is still important that we seek a cure.

Unfortunately, during the Reagan years, AIDS funding and HIV in general were ignored. From 1985 to 1990, research had been moving ahead by leaps and bounds; after the death of Rock Hudson money seemed to be more readily available. But it was suddenly halted by a lack of funds. AIDS must reemerge as a priority and must be given the necessary research-and-development money until proper treatment or a cure is found. AZT is being considered by some government officials as the HIV "cure," when it is in fact far from it.

In addition, although the FDA did relax its approval process of AZT, ddI, and ddC, the agency has once again put stringent demands on new HIV drugs. Its reasoning is that with the three treatments now approved and available, no other options are urgently needed. The truth is that the available drugs are not entirely effective, extremely toxic, and unusable as long-term treatments. All of us in the HIV community must pressure the FDA to allow new drugs to emerge and be approved at a faster rate.

Given the current limitations, though, what concrete developments are on the horizon?

The two most exciting drugs currently being tested are:

- TAT inhibitors
- and a vaccine called GP160, a treatment for people already infected

TAT INHIBITORS

TAT inhibitors, a new class of antiviral drugs, are promising for several reasons:

- First, TAT inhibitors are effective even in chronically infected cells. Macrophages and other cells besides T_4 cells become infected with HIV, causing dysfunction. TAT inhibitors would deactivate the virus in these cells as well as in T_4 cells. The current nucleoside analogues only stop HIV from reproducing, and reproduction occurs only in T_4 cells.
- Also, TAT inhibitors are less likely than other treatments to incur resistance.

TAT is a protein produced by HIV and used by the virus in the HIV-replication process. Early testing of this drug is extremely promising, not only in the treatment of HIV infection, but possibly also against PML, progressive multifocal leukoencephalopathy, an opportunistic infection for which there is currently no treatment.

Unfortunately, the development process of TAT inhibitors has been slow. Hoffmann–La Roche's drug RO-24-7429 is the first TAT inhibitor to have entered human testing. In animals, high doses of this drug cause kidney toxicity, and the drug seems to have complex pharmacokinetics—the processes governing the body's absorption and distribution of the drug. Trials for these drugs are continuing, but I believe we need to move forward more aggressively.

GP160

GP160, certainly the most promising of the HIV treatments, which works as an immune modulator, has been tested extensively. At the Eighth International AIDS Conference, many studies were presented on the effectiveness of this vaccine for people already infected with HIV. However, the drug has been tested only in people with high T4-cell counts. The reason for this is that researchers have wanted to test the drug against a placebo and have considered it unethical to test people with low T4 cells on a placebo-controlled study without using the currently approved antivirals, such as AZT.

Almost three years of research and data on this immune-restoring drug does not seem to be enough for the FDA to issue approval, and I personally wonder why. The drug has been shown to increase T cells significantly in people who are HIV-infected and stabilize them at T-cell counts of between 700 and 800 without any adverse effects. This is certainly one of the drugs I mean when I ask, "Why isn't it on the market yet?" Look for GP160 to emerge in the next couple of years as an extremely promising treatment.

HYPERICIN

As I mentioned in Chapter 8, hypericin is highly active in the test tube against HIV infection, but studies of an intravenous preparation of this drug have been slow and tedious. There is still hope that hypericin in an intravenous preparation might be an extremely effective antiviral, but oral preparations have yet to be proven effective. A recently developed 10-mg dose shows antiviral activity against CMV (see Chapter 8). At this writing, this dose is showing promise in preliminary tests against HIV.

COMPOUND Q

Mentioned in Chapter 10, Compound Q is an inexpensive anti-viral treatment that has been researched only by small community-based organizations. Because it is an inexpensive treatment, no large drug company has picked it up for development. There is more research on this treatment than on most HIV treatments, and it is currently available through buyers clubs; but it still requires more widespread testing and FDA approval. Following the publication of a conference abstract (PoB 3442) that chronicled dose-dependent changes in surrogate markers, testing on Compound Q has increased. Look for studies in your area by dialing 1-800-TRIALS-A.

ANGIOGENESIS INHIBITORS

This class of drugs stops the growth of tumors—it has shown effectiveness against Kaposi's sarcoma—by restricting the body's production of new blood vessels. Since tumors and KS need to produce new blood vessels to grow, these conditions virtually disappear when the body stops producing new blood vessels.

In research done by Paul Gallo, M.D., on the angiogenesis inhibitor SP-PG, there was dramatic improvement in KS lesions implanted in mice. For some reason, the development of this drug, SP-PG, has been delayed, but it is finally being mounted by Daiichi Pharmaceuticals. In addition to being a wonderful treatment for KS, this drug also shows promise as a treatment for tumors related to cancers, particularly breast cancer.

PASSIVE IMMUNIZATION

Passive immunization is the process by which HIV antibodies taken from healthy HIV-infected individuals are recirculated into less healthy HIV-infected people. This therapy not only looks extremely promising, but it is an organic product that is toxicity-free. I know of no reason that this treatment should not be used currently, given the existing data. Certainly, the theory of rebuilding an immune system by recirculating healthy antibodies is not only sound but has been proven for years by the use of gamma globulin. This treatment would work by supporting the immune system and using the body's natural defenses to control the HIV virus.

HemaCare Corporation of Los Angeles announced the preliminary analysis of its 12-month study of hyperimmune therapy (that is, passive immunization). HemaCare Corporation claimed the process improved survival, preserved T4 levels, and maintained immune competence. In an article in *AIDS Treatment News* (December 18, 1992), author Dave Gilden questioned the statistical analysis of HemaCare studies, citing some problems in data collection.

In any case, the low toxicity of this treatment should give it a priority status, but it has not received any such consideration. Due to the high cost of this treatment, researchers and insurance companies will demand extensive and concrete data before it will be approved.

There are a few doctors performing this procedure, which is totally legal. See Resource Guide.

566 C 80

This treatment will be on the market soon and will be a welcome addition for treating PCP pneumonia and, possibly, toxoplasmosis, since it is less toxic than current treatments for these illnesses.

D4T

This nucleoside analogue shows safety and efficacy and, as I mentioned in Chapter 10, is available in expanded-access programs. It will be available to the general public soon.

THREE-DRUG COMBINATION THERAPY

In February of 1993, the British journal *Nature* reported that Yung-Kang Chow, a Harvard Medical School student, combined AZT, ddI, and a third drug, either pyridinone or nevirapine, in a test tube and successfully stopped HIV's replication process. Prior to this, with the already-studied combinations of AZT and ddI, the viral replication process was slowed, but not stopped. The addition of the third drug seems to do the trick with the virus, for some reason, being able to mutate past the first and second drugs, but mutating into a harmless form at the third drug's intervention point. Needless to say, this is an exciting development, but the research is extremely preliminary. Human trials are set to begin in July and this is a process to watch. If it works in humans as well as in the test tube, this might be the treatment we've been waiting for. Still, many people are intolerant to AZT and ddI, so I remain cautiously hopeful.

SUMMARY

Many, many treatments are being developed for HIV infection. The Resource Guide lists three important directories for people interested in more information on experimental treatments. One is the 1-800-TRIALS-A number, which provides information on trials currently available to people. The other is the *AmFAR Directory*, an overview of all the latest documentation on all the treatments that have been tested for HIV infection. The last listing in the Resource Guide is the phone number for Project Inform, which will update any caller on current information by phone and mail.

As people involved in HIV infection, we must keep the pressure on the government, the FDA, and our local congresspeople to expand, explore, and continue to fund AIDS-treatment research.

CHAPTER 19

Keeping Current

The most important aspect of research literature is reader-friendliness. Often, journal articles that report original studies of treatments are filled with complex technical language, making them less than ideal for the lay reader. The best sources of information are periodicals that give overviews of a number of studies on different drugs that occurred in the last month or two-month period. As a rule, these surveys contain references to the original material, so you can track them down if you want to.

In this chapter, I survey the periodicals that I myself use to stay updated. I also describe others that could be useful to you in gathering treatment information. I have organized the periodicals into these categories:

• *Publications of community-based organizations.* These publications often report on drugs and alternatives being used or researched. Some community-based organizations, such as GMHC have their own treatment-specific periodicals. GMHC's *Treatment Issues* is devoted to medical treatment options, and sometimes alternative treatments, for HIV infection. Many of these publications are free.

• *Publications written for laypeople as well as medical professionals.* These publications contain technical information but are extremely reader-friendly in their writing style. Many contain excellent early information on treatment options. These periodicals are usually available to HIV+ people at reduced rates.

• *Professional journals for medical personnel.* These publications are sometimes technical, often very expensive, and sometimes completely out of the financial range of most laypeople.

• *Miscellaneous.* Hard-to-classify publications with their own particular contributions to make to the HIV literature.

I have included a description and pertinent information for each title in these categories. Often, one source will lead you to others, which means that this chapter actually represents a wealth of information. Still, I certainly do not claim that this or any other resource in this book is the be-all and end-all of resource directories. If you are just beginning to gather information on HIV infection, these materials are essential. Also, though they may overlap, these resources make a wonderful addition to any information you might already have collected.

By the way, if you actually *are* looking for the be-all and end-all of resource guides, I have the title for you:

• *AIDS: Information Sourcebook,* published by Oryx Press.

This resource guide is a state-by-state directory of AIDS organizations. In one 150-page section it lists a total of 994 agencies, the most comprehensive listing I've seen. In another, 50-page section, you'll find a bibliography of periodicals, brochures, pamphlets, books, and articles. A chronological recap of all the events that marked the progression of the HIV pandemic covers another 25 pages. This sourcebook is readily available by contacting Oryx Press. Write to:

Oryx Press
4041 North Central at Indian School Road
Suite 700
Phoenix, AZ 85012-3397
(800) 279-ORYX
Toll-free fax (800) 279-4663
Outside the U.S. call: (602) 265-2651; or fax: (602) 265-6250
Price: $39.95

The sourcebook seemed a little expensive to me at first, but it is finely produced and contains an extraordinary amount of information.

Below are two other sources of treatment-option information. These huge books are comprehensive, technical guides for physicians written in a style that is, for the most part, lay-reader-friendly:

1. *The AIDS Knowledge Base.* Edited by P. T. Cohen, M.D., Ph.D.; Merle A. Sande, M.D.; and Paul A. Volberding, M.D. (Waltham, Mass.: The Medical Publishing Group, Massachusetts Medical Society, 1990). To order, write to:

Massachusetts Medical Society
1440 Main Street
Waltham, MA 02154
(800) 843-6356
(617) 893-3800 (in Massachusetts)

2. *The Medical Management of AIDS.* Edited by Merle A. Sande and Paul A. Volberding (Philadelphia, Pa.: W. B. Saunders, 1990). To order, write to:

Harcourt Brace Jovanovich, Inc.
The Curtis Center
Independence Square West
Philadelphia, PA 19106

Although I find these resources extraordinarily useful, I'm hoping the publishers might be a little more sensitive to semantics in upcoming editions. The political aspects of HIV affect anyone who is professionally involved with the infection, and publishers with the potential to reach both HIV+ people and caregivers everywhere are certainly no exception. In the interest of raising consciousness generally, I think it's fair to point out that they occasionally use the word *AIDS* on the pages in their sourcebooks instead of *HIV infection,* and as we all know, *AIDS* was a term created by the Centers for Disease Control and Prevention (CDC) for the purpose of determining who would get federal benefits and who wouldn't. Many doctors use the term *HIV disease,* and supposedly that's a better choice than

HIV infection, but to me *disease* means *disease*—and HIV+ people are not diseased; they are simply infected, as we all are, with millions of microbes, viruses, and bacteria. In our time in history, it's important for all of us affected by the infection to be involved not only in the pricing of books on the subject, but in the careful and sensitive expression of information. Watchdogging the quality of the information circulating among us is related to our commitment to maintaining our dignity and insisting on being treated as the extremely significant people that we are.

Am I nitpicking? Not at all. Decisions made by publishers, by government agencies, by Congress, by drug companies affect *us*—and we need to speak out whenever we disagree with what we see. At this writing, for example, a bill is before Congress to stop free trade in the vitamin industry. I urge anyone I meet to write their senators and representatives to say they will not stand by and watch their health options narrowed any further. It's a matter of watching out for ourselves and each other.

PUBLICATIONS OF COMMUNITY-BASED ORGANIZATIONS

New York State Directory of AIDS/HIV Clinical Trials, published by AmFAR (American Foundation for AIDS Research). A vital part of any treatment library, this bilingual directory (English and Spanish) gives an overview of the clinical trial process, a listing of all drug trials in the tristate area (New York, Connecticut, New Jersey) and Philadelphia (where AmFAR is located), whom to contact about entering the trials, drug descriptions, and glossary. The directory is published four times a year and is free for HIV+ people.

To subscribe, contact:

Joseph Guimento
American Foundation for AIDS Research
733 Third Avenue
Twelfth Floor
New York, NY 10017-3204
(212) 682-7440

Also available through AmFAR is the *AmFAR Directory,* a comprehensive overview of the latest research for all HIV-treatment options and treatments for opportunistic infections. This is an essential directory for anyone dealing with HIV.

The Body Positive (New York). This monthly, grass-roots magazine combines a few articles on treatments with articles on emotional issues, letters, personals, announcements of events and lectures, and a Community Resource Guide, mostly limited to New York. Free to those who cannot afford a donation.

The Body Positive
2095 Broadway
Suite 306
New York, NY 10023
(212) 721-1619
Hot line: (212) 721-1346

CRIA Update. This small bulletin is published by Community Research Initiative on AIDS, an organization that does community-based drug trials (CRIA was responsible for the approval of the pentamidine inhalant). This bulletin has frequently published the latest results of drug trials CRIA has completed. It also announces drug trials in which CRIA is trying to enroll participants. CRIA deals with many alternative and complementary treatments, since such interventions lack drug company money for running trials. The bulletin is free.

Community Research Initiative on AIDS
31 West 26th Street
New York, NY 10010
(212) 889-1958
Fax: (212) 683-2197

Critical Path AIDS Project. This comprehensive, monthly grass-roots magazine comes out of Philadelphia. It covers HIV-related issues such as treatment options and emotional issues and contains a detailed resource guide for the Philadelphia area. Published in association with

The AIDS Library of Philadelphia
32 North 3rd Street
Philadelphia, PA 19106

(215) 922-5120
Fax: (215) 022-6762
Subscription: $50; $15 for PWAs on limited income.
Free for PWAs and HIV+s who cannot afford anything.

Critical Path Aids Project, Inc.
2062 Lombard Street
Philadelphia, PA 19146
(215) 545-2212

Digest: The Treatment and Data Digest. This is a weekly review of issues addressed by ACT UP's Treatment and Data Committee:

Mike Barr (212) 982-8206
Chris DeBlasit (212) 420-8432
Rich Lynn (212) 725-4689
Subscription price $40/year.
Make check payable to:

ACT UP/NY
155 East 31st Street
Suite 20L
New York, NY 10016

GMHC's *Treatment Issues.* This publication offers the latest information on alternative and mainstream treatments in easy-to-read articles with references. It is a must for anyone who wishes to keep up with the latest information. Published ten times a year, *Treatment Issues* is free to HIV+s who cannot afford to pay.

Suggested rates:
$30/individuals
$50/physicians and institutions
$60/foreign

Make checks payable to:
Gay Men's Health Crisis (GMHC)
Medical Information
129 West 20th Street
New York, NY 10011
(212) 337-3541

HEAL (Health Education AIDS Liaison). HEAL specializes in alternative therapies. The organization does not put out a periodical publication but a packet, called a HEAL packet, that covers a wide range of alternative treatments. The packet comes in two forms:

- a $6 packet, which contains extensive treatment information;
- a $30 packet, which describes all the studies available (and sometimes reprints them) along with the treatment information.

Remember: If you decide on an alternative intervention, thoroughly research the effectiveness of the treatment and then monitor yourself closely.

HEAL has weekly meetings in the New York City area.

HEAL
P.O. Box 1103
Old Chelsea Station
New York, NY 10013
(212) 674-HOPE

Notes from the Underground. This newsletter is published every other month by the PWA Health Group, a New York buyers club. It contains the latest information on the availability of unapproved drugs as well as other treatment information.

$35/individuals
$75/institutions and physicians
Sliding scale/low-income people
Make check payable to:

PWA Health Group
150 West 26th Street
Suite 201
New York, NY 10001
(212) 255-0520
Fax: (212) 255-2080

PI Perspective. This monthly magazine published by Project Inform provides extensive information on the latest treatments and

HIV-related issues. Project Inform also provides an indispensable hot-line service for people seeking information on treatment options. You can call the 800 number and ask for information about any treatment option. The staffer will answer your questions and/or mail you an information packet on a specific treatment or treatments.

Project Inform
1965 Market Street
Suite 220
San Francisco, CA 94103
National: (800) 822-7422
California: (800) 334-7422
San Francisco: (415) 558-9051

SIDA Ahora. This is the Hispanic sister magazine of *PWA Coalition Newsline* and a must for HIV+ Hispanic people. Each issue contains a great resource guide at the back.

PWA Coalition Newsline
31 West 26th Street
Fifth Floor
New York, NY 10010
(800) 828-3280

PROFESSIONAL PUBLICATIONS WITH A LAY READERSHIP

AIDS Treatment News. This excellent, readable compilation is published twice a month and provides the results from many different sources on HIV treatment options, both mainstream and alternative. This is another on the "must" list.

Subscriptions are:
$230/year for professionals
$115/year for nonprofit organizations
$100/year for individuals
$45/year or $24/6 months for people with financial
    difficulties
Subscription information: (800) TREAT-1-2

BETA: Bulletin of Experimental Treatments for AIDS. This bulletin contains brief, easy-to-read summaries of the latest information on treatment developments and other articles on HIV-related information. Published by the San Francisco AIDS Foundation four times a year. Subscriptions are:

$45/individuals
$95/institutions
Free to people in San Francisco

For subscription information:
Phone: (415) 863-2437
Fax: (415) 549-4342

Editorial office:
BETA
25 Van Ness Avenue
Suite 700
San Francisco, CA 94102

CDC AIDS Weekly. This weekly magazine, published by the Centers for Disease Control and Prevention, reports the latest findings on HIV treatments. Short, easy-to-read reports on the latest studies make this, in my opinion, the best publication on HIV treatment options and on recent developments in HIV research. The only drawback is the price:

$789/year in the United States, Canada, and Mexico
$893/year in all other countries

Call for a free sample copy or to order a subscription;
800-633-4931
or write:
CDC AIDS Weekly
Subscription Office
P.O. Box 830409
Birmingham, AL 35283-0409

MMWR (Morbidity and Mortality Weekly Report). This is a weekly publication of the Centers for Disease Control and Prevention. It often covers HIV topics and clinical issues of HIV infection—for example, recommendations for prevention of transmission in health-care settings or revision of the CDC Surveillance Case definition of AIDS. Individual supplements on HIV topics are available through:

National AIDS Clearinghouse
(800) 458-5231

Subscriptions are available from:
Superintendent of Documents
U.S. Government Printing Office
Washington, DC 20402-9371
(202) 783-3238

Also available by subscription through:
Massachusetts Medical Society Publications
$69/year first-class mail
$46/year second-class mail

Write to:
MMS Publications
GSPO Box 9120
Waltham, MA 02254
(800) 843-6356 (outside Massachusetts)
(617) 893-3800 (in Massachusetts)

PROFESSIONAL JOURNALS

Journal of Acquired Immune Deficiency Syndrome. This monthly journal prints studies on treatments and other HIV-related issues. It can get extremely technical and is recommended for medical professionals only.

Raven Press
1185 Avenue of the Americas
New York, NY 10036
(212) 930-9604

AIDS Patient Care. This publication often translates complex medical language into simple, readable articles. It is informative and *extremely* mainstream.

Rates are per volume of six issues:
$69/USA
$104/foreign

Make checks payable to:
Liebert Enterprises, Inc.

Mail to:
Mary Ann Liebert, Inc.
1651 Third Avenue
New York, NY 10128
Attention: Subscription Department
(212) 289-2300

MISCELLANEOUS

National AIDS Clearinghouse. This public health service distributes *free* videotapes, posters, brochures, and fact sheets. It also provides a service called NAC On-Line. You log in with your computer and reach a bulletin board or data base containing listings for more than 14,000 service providers throughout the world. This is *too much!*

Phone 9 A.M. to 7 P.M. Eastern time: (800) 458-5231

AIDS Surveillance Update. The New York City Department of Health publishes this free quarterly report of the latest data on AIDS incidences. Most of the data is New York City–specific, but there is an overview of U.S. cases.

Call:
(212) 566-8906 or (212) 566-7793
or write:
New York City Department of Health
Office of AIDS Surveillance
346 Broadway
Room 706, Box 44
New York, NY 10013

Hazelden Publishing Group, publisher of educational materials. Hazelden publishes a range of educational materials. The company concentrates on substance abuse but publishes many books and pamphlets about HIV infection. The materials are oriented toward the emotional experience of the infection.

Call for a brochure:
(800) 328-9000 (United States, Canada, and Virgin Islands)
(612) 257-4010 (outside the United States and Canada)
Fax: (612) 257-1331

NDRI Training Institute. This institute has some of the best training programs on HIV infection I have ever attended. The institute is located in New York City, but its programs are held throughout New York State. Call or write for information, prices, and schedule:

NDRI
11 Beach Street
Second Floor
New York, NY 10013
(212) 966-8700

A Resource Guide

Services and resources throughout the United States and Europe are constantly changing, so it's impossible to provide an exhaustive or definitive list of HIV-related resources here. But this guide will get you started in finding the resources in your area. One find will lead you to another, and this pattern of networking—especially with other HIV-infected people—will undoubtedly lead you to the person, treatment, book, agency, service, or product you need.

I'm taking the liberty of listing myself as the first resource. Call me about consultations and distribution information for Super Blue-Green Algae.

NICK SIANO'S OFFICE

(800) 769-HEAL or 769-4325
From within New York State: (718) 376-8824

ACUPUNCTURE

Dr. Frank Lipman (212) 255-1800
Jacqueline Haught (212) 769-6445

DRUG TRIAL INFORMATION

(800) TRIALS-A
Monday through Friday, 9:00 AM through 7:00 PM, EST
TTY/TDD: (800) 243-7012

AmFAR Directory and *New York State AIDS/HIV Clinical Trials
Directory* (covering Connecticut, New Jersey, and Philadelphia)
American Foundation for AIDS Research
733 Third Avenue
Twelfth Floor
New York, NY 10017
(212) 682-7440

NATIONAL AIDS CLEARINGHOUSE
(800) 458-5231

GOVERNMENT AGENCIES

CENTERS FOR DISEASE CONTROL AND PREVENTION (CDC)
(800) 342-2437

FOOD AND DRUG ADMINISTRATION (FDA)
5600 Fischers Lane
Rockville, MD 20857
Director: Dr. David Kessler
(301) 443-1544

HIV LIBRARIES

HEALING ALTERNATIVES FOUNDATION
Treatment & Resource Library
1748 Market Street
San Francisco, CA 94102
(415) 626-4053

PEOPLE WITH AIDS COALITION—DADE
AIDS Library of South Florida
175 NE 36th Street
Miami, FL 33137
(305) 537-6010

NEW YORK CITY AIDS LIBRARY
New York City Department of Health
(212) 788-4280

AIDS LIBRARY OF PHILADELPHIA
32 North 3rd Street
Philadelphia, PA 19106
(215) 922-5120

HIV SPECIALIST

DR. PAUL CURTIS BELLMAN (212) 645-0161

LISTINGS OF NATIONAL AIDS AGENCIES

AIDS: Information Sourcebook, 1991–92
Oryx Press
4041 North Central Avenue at Indian School Road
Suite 700
Phoenix, AZ 85012-3397
(800) 279-ORYX
Toll-free fax: (800) 279-4663
Outside the U.S. call: (602) 265-2651; or fax: (602) 265-6250
Price: $39.95

National Directory of AIDS Care
Richards Publishing Company
4903 Calle Carinon NE
Albuquerque, NM 87111-2962
(505) 271-2159

NUTRITIONAL CONSULTATIONS

LAURA LANDON, M.S., R.D. (718) 945-6175

PASSIVE IMMUNIZATION

DR. GARY BLICK (203) 622-1118

TREATMENT INFORMATION SERVICES

PROJECT INFORM
From San Francisco: (415) 558-9051
From California: (800) 334-7422
From all other states: (800) 822-7422

Project Inform is the most important source of HIV-therapy information in the country. Call these numbers and ask the person who answers to mail you fact sheets and articles on specific HIV-related issues. Volunteers take the calls and sometimes lend their personal opinions to the information, so you're better off asking for a mailing to read the material and make up your own mind.

PWA COALITION HOT LINE
(800) 828-8380
PWA, in New York, provides a service similar to Project Inform.

GAY MEN'S HEALTH CRISIS (GMHC) HOT LINE
(212) 807-6655
This group provides a wide range of services.

SPIRITUAL SUPPORT, FREE MASSAGE, OTHER SUPPORT SERVICES

MANHATTAN CENTER FOR LIVING (212) 533-3550
LOS ANGELES CENTER FOR LIVING (213) 850-0877
FRIENDS IN DEED (212) 925-2009

VENDORS AND BUYERS CLUBS FOR ALTERNATIVE AND MAINSTREAM THERAPIES

ESTROFF PHARMACY
Scott Berliner
138 2nd Avenue
New York, NY 10003
(800)-9-ESTROFF or (212) 254-7760

Contact Estroff Pharmacy to buy a wide range of alternative and mainstream therapies, including Composition A, Enhance, NAC, phyllmartin, Ester C, and most of the other treatments and pharmaceuticals discussed in the book. Estroff's will charge your phone order to your credit card and mail it to you.

The following buyers clubs carry therapies not yet approved by the FDA but readily available and shipped from other countries. Call the clubs for listings of products and prices. These groups have internal quality-control procedures and are believed to be sound regarding the procurement, testing, and distribution of drugs. PWA Health Group in New York City has a particularly good reputation regarding quality-control standards.

Arizona

PAACT BUYERS CLUB/PWA COALITION
Tucson, Arizona
(602) 770-1710

California

HEALING ALTERNATIVES
San Francisco, California
(415) 626-2316

District of Columbia

CARL VOGEL FOUNDATION
District of Columbia
(202) 289-4898

DC BUYERS CLUB (DCBC)
District of Columbia
(202) 232-5494

Florida

PWA HEALTH ALLIANCE
Ft. Lauderdale, Florida
(800) 447-9242

PWA HEALTH ALLIANCE
Oakland Park, Florida
(305) 568-3001

AIDS MANASOTA
Sarasota, Florida
(813) 954-6011

Georgia

ATLANTA BUYERS CLUB
Atlanta, Georgia
(404) 874-4845

Illinois

CHICAGO BUYERS CLUB
Chicago, Illinois
(312) 509-5127

New York

PWA HEALTH GROUP
New York, New York
(212) 255-0520

DIRECT AIDS ALTERNATIVE INFORMATION RESOURCES (DAAIR)
New York, New York
(212) 689-8140

Texas

DBC ALTERNATIVES
Dallas, Texas
(214) 528-4460

VISITING NURSE SERVICES

VISITING NURSE ASSOCIATION
Houston, Texas
For AIDS team, pharmacy, and IV preparations in the home by
visiting nurses: (713) 796-1166
For national referrals: (800) 375-6877

VISITING NURSE ASSOCIATION OF MILWAUKEE
(414) 327-2295

VISITING NURSE SERVICE OF NEW YORK
(212) 714-9250

VISITING NURSE ASSOCIATION OF SAN FRANCISCO
Intake: (415) 431-4071
Evenings and weekends: (415) 861-4815
TTY/TDD: (415) 552-8349

KIMBERLY QUALITY CARE (LOS ANGELES)
(213) 650-1800
See also your local yellow pages.

COMMUNITY-BASED ORGANIZATIONS

This listing covers diverse groups—coalitions, task forces, and
other local organizations. Coalitions usually disseminate information on support groups, medical personnel, and treatment
options. Task forces are usually associated with local government.
Also, ACT UP (AIDS Coalition to Unleash Power), which has
local chapters in many cities, is the most successful, creative, and
influential AIDS activist organization. Contact the local ACT UP
group in your city for more information. The main characteristic
these groups share is that they all make referrals.

Alabama

| Birmingham | AIDS Task Force of Alabama | (205) 326-0628 Hot line |
| Huntsville | AIDS Action Coalition | (205) 533-2437 |

Alaska

| Anchorage | AIDS Network | (907) 343-6872 |

Arizona

| Phoenix | Arizona AIDS Information | (602) 234-2752 Hot line |
| | Arizona AIDS Project, Inc. | (602) 420-9396 Hot line |

Arkansas

| Little Rock | Arkansas AIDS Foundation | (501) 663-7833 |

California

Long Beach	Being Alive Long Beach	(310) 495-3422
Los Angeles	AIDS Project Los Angeles	(800) 922-2437 Hot line
	Multi Language	(800) 922-2438 Hot line
	TDD	(800) 553-2437 Hot line
	Spanish Language	(800) 400-7432 Hot line
Redondo Beach	Being Alive South Bay	(310) 544-8312
San Diego	Being Alive San Diego	(619) 291-1400
San Francisco	San Francisco AIDS Foundation	(415) 863-AIDS Hot line
San Mateo	San Mateo AIDS Network	(415) 573-2588

Colorado

| Denver | Colorado AIDS Project (CAP) | (303) 830-AIDS Hot line |
| Denver | PWA Coalition of Colorado | (303) 837-8214 |

Connecticut

Milford	PWA Coalition of Connecticut	(203) 249-6160
New Haven	AIDS Project New Haven (APNH) M–F 9–5	(203) 624-0947
	M–F 6:30 AM–9 PM	(203) 624-2437 Hot line

Delaware

Wilmington	AIDS Program Office (APO)	(302) 995-8582
		(302) 995-8681
		(302) 995-8653

District of Columbia

	The Positive Woman	(202) 898-0372

Florida

Broward County	PWA Coalition	(305) 565-9119
Clearwater	PWA Coalition Pinellas	(813) 449-2437
Coconut Grove	Cure AIDS Now	(305) 375-0400
Dade County	People With Aids Coalition—Dade	(305) 573-6010
Gainesville	North Central Florida AIDS Network (NCFAN)	(904) 372-4370 or (800) 824-6745
Jacksonville	PWA Coalition	(904) 398-9292 or (800) 851-1128
Miami	Body Positive	(305) 576-1111
Palm Beach	PWA Coalition	(407) 697-8033
Tampa Bay	PWA Coalition Tampa Bay	(813) 238-2887

Georgia

Atlanta	AIDS Atlanta	(404) 876-9940 Hot line
	National Association of PWA's Atlanta Chapter (NAPWA)	(404) 874-7926

Hawaii

Honolulu	Life Foundation/The AIDS Foundation of Hawaii	(808) 971-2437

Idaho

Boise	Idaho AIDS Foundation	(208) 345-2277

Illinois

Chicago	AIDS Foundation of Chicago (AFC)	(312) 642-3763
	Chicago Women's AIDS Project (CWAP)	(312) 271-2070

Indiana

Indianapolis	PWA Coalition	(317) 636-2134 Hot line
		(317) 637-2720

Iowa

Davenport	Quad City AIDS Coalition	(319) 324-8638

Kansas

Topeka	Topeka AIDS Project	(913) 232-3100

Kentucky

Newport	Northern Kentucky AIDS Task Force	(606) 341-4264

Louisiana

Alexandria	Central Louisiana AIDS Support Services	(318) 442-1010 Hot line
		(800) 444-7993
New Orleans	PWA Coalition	(504) 945-4500
		(504) 944-2437 Hot line
	Louisiana only	(800) 992-4379

Maine

Portland	The AIDS Project, Inc. (TAP)	(207) 775-1267 or (800) 851-AIDS Hot line
	PWA Coalition	(207) 773-8500

Maryland

Baltimore	PWA Coalition of Baltimore	(301) 625-1677

Massachusetts

Boston	Community Research Initiative	(617) 424-1524
Provincetown	Provincetown Positive	(508) 487-3998

Michigan

Grand Rapids	PWA Coalition Western Michigan	(616) 363-7689
	Grand Rapids AIDS Resource Center	(616) 459-9177

Minnesota

Minneapolis	The Aliveness Project Center For Living	(612) 822-3016 Hot line
	Minnesota AIDS Project	(612) 870-7773

Missouri

Saint Joseph	HIV/AIDS Coordinator	(816) 271-4684 Hot line
St. Louis	St. Louis Effort for AIDS	(314) 367-8400 Hot line

Montana

Missoula	Missoula AIDS Council	(406) 523-4775

Nebraska

Omaha	Nebraska AIDS Project	(402) 342-4233
		(800) 782-AIDS Hot line

Nevada

Reno	Nevada AIDS Foundation	(702) 329-AIDS

New Hampshire

Manchester	New Hampshire AIDS Foundation (NHAF)	(603) 623-0710

New Jersey

Atlantic City	South Jersey AIDS Alliance	(609) 348-2437 or (800) 432-AIDS
Bergenfield	PWA Coalition of New Jersey	(201) 944-6670
Collingswood	AIDS Coalition of Southern New Jersey	(609) 854-7578
New Brunswick	Hyacinth Foundation AIDS Project	(201) 246-0204 or (800) 433-0254

New Mexico

Albuquerque	New Mexico AIDS Services	(505) 984-0911 Hot line

New York

Albany	AIDS Institute	(800) 541-AIDS (800) 542-2437 Hot line
Bronx	Bronx AIDS Services	(800) 334-3477 Hot line (212) 295-5605
Brooklyn	Brooklyn AIDS Task Force	(718) 638-2437 Hot line
Flushing	AIDS Center of Queens County (ACQC)	(718) 896-2500

Long Island	Long Island Association for AIDS Care, Inc. (LIAAC)	(516) 385-AIDS
Manhattan	Body Positive	(212) 721-1346 Hot line
	Gay Men's Health Crisis	(212) 807-6655 Hot line
	PWA Coalition	(800) 828-3280
		(212) 532-0568

North Carolina

| Asheville | Western North Carolina AIDS Project (WNCAP) | (704) 252-7489 |

North Dakota

| Bismarck | AIDS Advisory Council | (701) 224-2378 |
| | *North Dakota only* | (800) 472-2180 Hot line |

Ohio

| Columbus | Columbus AIDS Task Force (CATF) | (614) 488-2437 |
| | *Ohio only* | (800) 332-AIDS |

Oklahoma

| Oklahoma City | Oasis Resource Center/ Oasis Foundation | (405) 525-2437 Hot line |

Oregon

| Portland | Portland Cascade AIDS Project, Inc. (CAP) | (503) 223-AIDS |
| | *Oregon only* | (800) 777-AIDS |

Pennsylvania

| Philadelphia | ActionAIDS | (215) 981-0088 |

Rhode Island

| Providence | Rhode Island Project/ AIDS (The Project) | (401) 831-5522 |
| | | (800) 726-3010 Hot line |

South Carolina

Columbia	South Carolina AIDS Task Force	(803) 734-5482
	South Carolina only	(800) 322-2437 Hot line

South Dakota

Pierre	South Dakota Department of Health/AIDS Program	(605) 773-3364
	South Dakota only	(800) 592-1861

Tennessee

Nashville	NAPWA Nashville	(615) 385-1510

Texas

Dallas	PWA Coalition	(214) 941-0523

Utah

Ogden	Northern Wasatch AIDS Coalition (NWAC)	(801) 627-3533

Vermont

Brattleboro	Vermont PWA Coalition	(802) 257-9277

Washington

Seattle	Health Information Network	(206) 784-5655

West Virginia

Morgantown	Friends Who Care	(304) 292-9000

Wisconsin

Milwaukee	PLWA of Milwaukee	(414) 273-1991

Wyoming

Casper	Wyoming AIDS Project	(307) 237-7833

Puerto Rico

San Juan	Fundacíon SIDA de Puerto Rico	(809) 782-9600

Canada
British Columbia

Vancouver	Vancouver AIDS Society (AIDS Vancouver)	(604) 687-2437 Hot line

Manitoba

Winnipeg	Village Clinic Inc.	(204) 453-0045

Ontario

Toronto	AIDS Committee of Toronto (ACT)	(416) 926-0063
	TTY/TDD	(416) 926-8295

Saskatchewan

Regina	AIDS Regina	(306) 525-0902 Hot line

England

London	Body Positive	071-373-9124 Help-line

BOOKS

This book list was compiled by Michael Miles and is reprinted
with his permission. One particularly excellent source for books
on spirituality, healing, and alternative medicine is:

East/West Bookstore
78 Fifth Avenue
New York, NY 10011
(212) 243-5994

Beginners

If you are just beginning to explore the idea of holistic healing, these books might serve as the starting point you have been looking for. All of them offer hope, insights, and encouragement.

Alive and Well: A Path of Healing in a Time of HIV by Peter Henderickson (New York: Irvington, 1990).

Beyond AIDS by George R. Melton (San Francisco: Brotherhood Press, 1988).

Discover the Power Within You by Eric Butterworth (San Francisco: Harper San Francisco, 1989).

Healing AIDS Naturally by Laurence E. Badgley (Foster City, Calif.: Human Energy Press, 1987).

How to Meditate: A Guide to Self-Discovery by Lawrence LeShan (New York: Bantam, 1984).

Living in the Light by Shakti Gawain (San Rafael, Calif.: New World Library, 1986).

Love, Medicine and Miracles by Bernie S. Siegel (New York: HarperCollins, 1990).

The Prescription for Nutritional Healing by James F. Balch and Phyllis Balch (Wayne, N.J.: Avery Publishing, 1990).

Who Dies by Stephen Levine (New York: Doubleday, 1989).

You Can Heal Your Life by Louise L. Hay (Carson, Calif.: Hay House, 1987).

You Can't Afford the Luxury of a Negative Thought by John-Roger and Peter McWilliams (New York: Bantam, 1991).

Death Awareness

Some—not all—people fear death and are even wary of reading about it. Although the books listed here may have the word *death* in the title, all of them are actually about living and appreciating

life to the fullest. If you are fearful, one of these books might help
to allay your anxiety.

Grief Recovery Handbook by John W. James and Frank Cherry (New
    York: HarperCollins, 1989).
Death: The Final Stage of Growth by Elisabeth Kübler-Ross (New
    York: Prentice-Hall, 1975).
Healing into Life and Death by Stephen Levine (New York: Double-
    day, 1989).
The Light Beyond by Raymond Moody, Jr. (New York: Bantam,
    1988).
Living with Death and Dying by Elisabeth Kübler-Ross (New York:
    Macmillan, 1982).
Meetings at the Edge by Stephen Levine (New York: Doubleday,
    1984).
Who Dies by Stephen Levine (New York: Doubleday, 1989).

Healing

These books focus on specific healing approaches. Some deal
with the balance of body, mind, and spirit, and all explore the
effects of the mind on health and well-being.

Anatomy of an Illness as Perceived by the Patient by Norman Cousins
    (New York: Bantam, 1983).
Ayurveda: The Science of Self-Healing by Vasant Lad (Wilmot, Wis.:
    Lotus Light, 1990).
Creating Health by Deepak Chopra (New York: Houghton Mifflin,
    1991).
Heal Your Body by Louise L. Hay (Carson, Calif.: Hay House,
    1988).
Healing Power of Humor by Allen Klein (Carson, Calif.: Hay
    House, 1988).
Peace, Love & Healing by Bernie S. Siegel (New York: Walker,
    1990).
Psychoimmunity and the Healing Process by Jason Serinus (Berkeley,
    Calif.: Celestial Arts, 1990).
Quantum Healing by Deepak Chopra (New York: Bantam, 1990).
You Can Heal Your Life by Louise L. Hay (Carson, Calif.:
    1987).

Herbs

To get the full benefit of Chinese herbs as a healing supplement, you need to know how they work with respect to body, mind, and spirit. You'll find these books to be valuable resources.

The Healing Herbs by Michael Castleman (Emmeas, Pa.: Rodale, 1991).

Planetary Herbology by Michael Tierra (Wilmot, Wis.: Lotus Light, 1988).

Holistic Overview

These books cover a wide range of holistic topics, from acupuncture to Zen, as they relate to HIV infection.

Alive and Well: A Path of Healing in a Time of HIV by Peter Henderickson (New York: Irvington, 1990).

Back to Eden by Jethro Kloss (Loma Linda, Calif.: Back to Eden Books Publishing Company, 1989).

Conquering AIDS Now by Gregory Scott and Bianca Leonardo (New York: Warner Books, 1987).

Healing AIDS Naturally by Laurence E. Badgley (Foster City, Calif.: Human Energy Press, 1987).

Holistic Protocol for the Immune System by Gregory J. Scott (Palm Springs, Calif.: Tree of Life Publications, 1992).

Our Healing Birthright by Andrew M. Cort (Rochester, Vt.: Inner Traditions, 1990).

Immunity

More and more books on the immune system are appearing. The more we learn the more obvious it becomes that everything we think, do, and feel is filtered through that system to affect our physical health.

AIDS, Macrobiotics, and Natural Immunity by Michio Kushi and Martha C. Cotrell (Briarcliff Manor, N.Y.: Japan Publications USA, 1989).

Natural Immunity: Insights on Diet and AIDS by Noboru B. Muramoto (Oroville, Calif.: George Ohsawa Macrobiotic Foundation, 1988).

Super Immunity by Paul Pearsall (New York: Fawcett, 1988).
Understanding Your Immune System by Eve Potts and Marion Molla (New York: Avon, 1986).

Meditation

Prayer is talking to God; meditation is listening to God talking to you. You are unlikely to find a more effective path to stress reduction, clarity of thought, peace of mind, and general well-being than some form of meditation. These books will give you an idea of how to get started.

Color of Light by Perry Tillerass (San Francisco: Harper San Francisco, 1988).
Creative Visualization by Shakti Gawain (San Rafael, Calif.: New World Library, 1978).
Going Within: A Guide to Self-Discovery by Lawrence LeShan (New York: Bantam, 1984).
Gradual Awakening by Stephen Levine (New York: Doubleday, 1989).
How to Meditate: A Guide to Self-Discovery by Lawrence LeShan (New York: Bantam, 1984).
Inner Health by Nevill Drury (Wayne, N.J.: Avery Publishing, 1985).
The Joy of Meditation by Jack Addington and Cornelia Addington (Marina del Ray, Calif.: DeVorss, 1979).
Love Your Body by Louise L. Hay (Carson, Calif.: Hay House, 1989).
Quiet Mind: Techniques for Transforming Stress by John Harvey (Honesdale, Pa.: Himalayan Publications, 1989).

HIV

This group of books covers a wide range of topics related to HIV infection, from alternative therapies to the politics of AIDS to challenging the premise that HIV exists at all.

AIDS: The HIV Myth by Jad Adams (New York: St. Martin's, 1989).
AIDS and Syphilis: The Hidden Link by Harris L. Coulter (Washington D.C.: Center for Empirical Medicine, 1987).
AIDS Treatment News by John S. James (Berkeley, Calif.: Celestial Arts, 1989).

Complete Book of Acupuncture by Stephen Chang (Berkeley, Calif.:
Celestial Arts, 1976).

The Great AIDS Hoax by T. C. Fry (New York: Gordon Press,
1992).

Oxygen Therapies by Ed McCabe (Morrisville, N.Y.: Energy Publications, 1989).

Poison by Prescription: The AZT Story by John Lauritsen (New York:
Pagan Press, 1990).

Nutrition

More than half the cancer in this country is directly related to
what we eat! When the immune system is compromised by the
presence of pesticides, preservatives, chemicals, and additives,
the HIV virus thrives. It's impossible to overstate the need for
eating natural, whole, organic foods.

Food and Healing by Annemarie Colbin (New York: Ballantine,
1986).

Hippocrates Diet and Health Program by Ann Wigmore (Wayne,
N.J.: Avery, 1984).

The Prescription for Nutritional Healing by James F. Balch and Phyllis Balch (Wayne, N.J.: Avery, 1990).

The Self-Healing Cookbook by Kristina Turner (Grass Valley, Calif.:
Earthtones, 1988).

Surviving with AIDS by C. Callaway and Catherine Whitney (Boston: Little, Brown, 1991).

The Vegetarian Handbook by Gary Null (New York: St. Martin's,
1988).

Personal Transformation

These inspiring books tell the true stories of people who met
their health challenges and experienced miraculous results.

Beyond AIDS by George R. Melton (San Francisco: Brotherhood
Press, 1988).

Dancing in the Light by Shirley MacLaine (New York: Bantam,
1985).

Out on a Limb by Shirley MacLaine (New York: Bantam, 1986).

Roger's Recovery from AIDS by Bob Owen (Pacific Palisades, Calif.:
Davar, 1987).

Surviving AIDS by Michael Callen (New York: HarperCollins, 1991).

Why I Survive AIDS by Niro Markoff and Paul Duffy (New York: Avon, 1991).

Self-Empowerment

If you can change your mind; that is, your thoughts about yourself and the world, you can change *anything*. Healing begins in the mind, which in turn affects the immune system.

AIDS and the Healer Within by Nick Bamford (Woodstock, N.Y.: Amethyst Books, 1988).

AIDS Book: Creating a Positive Approach by Louise L. Hay (Carson, Calif.: Hay House, 1988).

AIDS: The Ultimate Challenge by Elisabeth Kübler-Ross (New York: Macmillan, 1988).

Head First: The Biology of Hope by Norman Cousins (New York: Viking Penguin, 1990).

In the Absence of Angels by Elizabeth Glaser (New York: Berkley, 1991).

Living with AIDS by Tom O'Connor (Newbury Park, Calif.: Corwin, 1986).

Love, Medicine & Miracles by Bernie S. Siegel (New York: HarperCollins, 1990).

Notes on Living Until We Say Goodbye by Lon G. Nungesser (New York: St. Martin's, 1989).

The Power Is Within You by Paul Reed (Berkeley, Calif.: Celestial Arts, 1990).

Trusting the Healer Within by Nick Bamford (Woodstock, N.Y.: Amethyst Books, 1989).

You Can't Afford the Luxury of a Negative Thought by John-Roger and Peter McWilliams (New York: Bantam, 1991).

Spirituality

We are all spiritual beings. If we look at the world with an open mind, we will see that all roads lead within. It is there that we will find God, the Universe, a Higher Power, the Light, or whatever peace you are looking for under whatever name you attach to it. Love is our guide; truth is our destination.

A Course in Miracles (Tiburon, Calif.: Foundation for Inner Peace, 1992).

Discover the Power Within You by Eric Butterworth (San Francisco: Harper San Francisco, 1988).

Emmanuel's Book by Pat Rodegast and Judith Stanton (New York: Bantam, 1985).

Emmanuel's Book 2: The Choice of Love by Pat Rodegast and Judith Stanton (New York: Bantam, 1989).

For the Love of God by various authors (San Rafael, Calif.: New World Library, 1990).

God Never Fails by Mary L. Kupferle (Marina del Ray, Calif.: DeVorss, 1983).

I Am by Jean Klein (Santa Barbara, Calif.: Third Millennium, 1989).

Living in the Light by Shakti Gawain (San Rafael, Calif.: New World Library, 1987).

The Miracle of Mindfulness by Thich Nhat Hanh (San Rafael, Calif.: New World Library, 1988).

Quiet Moments with God by Joseph Murphy (Marina del Ray, Calif.: DeVorss, 1958).

Reflections in the Light by Shakti Gawain (San Rafael, Calif.: New World Library).

A Return to Love by Marianne Williamson (New York: Harper-Collins, 1992).

Return of the Rishi by Deepak Chopra (New York: Houghton Mifflin, 1989).

Glossary

Acupressure: A method of massage in which pressure is applied to acupuncture points with the fingers.

Acupuncture: Ancient Chinese medicine provides the knowledge for this healing technique in which extremely thin needles are placed in different acupuncture points on the body to promote the body's natural ability to heal.

Adjunct therapies: Treatment interventions used to supplement mainstream medical treatments.

Affirmation: A self-healing process in which positive statements are repeated over and over.

Aggressive: Used to describe healing techniques that have significant side effects or toxicity but get quick results.

AIDS: Acquired immunodeficiency syndrome.

Alternative therapies: Treatments, usually natural and nontoxic, used to promote healing.

Antibodies: Cells created by the immune system to neutralize infectious agents (toxins) within the body.

Antiviral: Treatments that control or stop a given virus.

Apoptosis: A process by which the body eliminates cells no longer useful.

ARC: AIDS-related complex.

Asymptomatic: Without symptoms.

B cells: The white blood cells in the immune system that make antibodies.

Baseline bloodwork: The bloodwork results you begin with and measure later results against.

Bloodwork: Lab results that measure properties and cells within the blood system.

Brand names: Registered Trademark names companies use to identify products or drugs.

CD4 cells: White blood cells or immune system cells that orchestrate immune response.

Cell: A basic unit in the structure of living matter or within the bloodstream.

Centers for Disease Control and Prevention (CDC): The government agency that monitors and develops policies for infectious diseases.

Clinical trials: The process that identifies drug efficacy.

Cofactors: Elements that influence the progression of a condition and may increase the likelihood of illness.

Complementary treatments: Treatments that add benefit to a given treatment regimen.

Definitive diagnosis: A diagnosis made by actual proof of the existence of a virus, bacteria, or toxin; performed by taking a culture or biopsy, or other invasive procedures.

Diagnostic procedure: The method used to diagnose a given condition.

DNA: A complex protein that carries genetic information.

Docking arms: The "hooks" that protrude from the HIV virus and enable it to attach to, and infect, cells.

Dormancy: The period an organism in the body is not producing any ill effects.

Efficacy: Capacity of a treatment to produce results.

Enzyme: A substance in the body that creates chemical reactions.

Food and Drug Administration (FDA): The government agency that tests and licenses drugs.

Generic names: Drug names used to identify substances that are not identified with or trademarked by any particular drug company.

Genetic code: The instructions within a cell that make it function.

Glutathione: A substance composed of three amino acids that helps protect cells from damage caused by oxidizing or cleansing agents in the blood.

Gp-120 (glyco protein 120): The scientific name for the "docking arms" of the HIV virus.

Helper cell: *See* T4 cell.

Herbology: The practice of prescribing herbs for healing.

HIV infection (disease): The process and resulting effects of the body's long-term interaction with the HIV virus.

Holistic treatments: Substances or regimens, usually nontoxic, that alternative or "natural" practitioners use.

Homeopathy: A treatment process that prescribes extremely small doses of substances that actually create the very symptoms of the disease which you are seeking treatment for; the theoretical belief is that these small exposures will stimulate a vaccine-type immunity.

Host cell: The infected cell.

Immune modulators: Treatment interventions that stimulate or build immune-system cells.

Immune response: The body's reaction to toxins that protects it from illness.

Immune system: Cells in the body that protect it from illness caused by infectious agents.

In vitro: In the test tube.

In vivo: In the body.

Infection: The process by which an infectious agent (virus, bacteria, toxin) multiplies and causes ill effects within the body.

Intramuscular injections: Drugs delivered into muscle tissue through a needle and syringe.

Macrophage: The white blood cell or immune system cell that activates the immune system and ultimately eliminates the neutralized infectious agent.

Mainstream treatments: Drugs that have been approved by the FDA and are prescribed by doctors for a given condition.

Markers: Lab results or symptom observation used to measure a treatment's effectiveness.

Nucleus: The core of a cell.

Off-label prescriptions: The practice of prescribing FDA-approved drugs for symptoms or diseases other than those cited by the FDA approval.

OI: Opportunistic infection.

OI treatments: Substances or regimens used to cure or stop the progression of an opportunistic infection.

Presumptive diagnosis: Diagnostic procedure in which the practitioner assumes an infection is present from symptom observation and any other monitoring techniques that do not include actually seeing or performing a culture or biopsy of the virus, bacteria, or toxin.

Primary prophylaxis: Treatments given to prevent infections when lab results indicate patient is at high risk of developing a particular infection.

Progression: The process of disease advancement.

Prophylactic treatments: Substances given to prevent disease.

Retrovirus: A class of viruses that replicate from RNA, as opposed to most viruses, which replicate from DNA.

Reverse transcriptase: A retroviral enzyme that is capable of copying RNA into DNA, essential for HIV replication.

RNA: A complex protein that carries genetic information.

Secondary prophylaxis: Treatments given to prevent recurrence of a disease after the patient has had the disease and has been cured.

Seroconversion: When the HIV-antibody blood test changes from negative to positive.

Spectrum of infection: The different stages of disease progression.

Symptomatic: The development of symptoms of HIV infection.

Synctium: A dysfunctional clump of cells, which can be caused by HIV.

Syndrome: A group of symptoms and/or diseases that are characteristic of a specific condition.

T4 cell (CD4 cell; T cell): A white blood cell or immune-system cell that moderates the immune response.

T8 cell (suppressor cell): A white blood cell or immune-system cell that ends an immune response.

Titer: A measurement of the volume or concentration of a particular element in a given solution.

Toxicity: The extent, quality, or degree to which a substance or treatment is harmful to the body.

Transmission agent: The substance that transfers a given element.

Viral core: The nucleus, or center, of a virus.

Viral progression: The process of viral advancement, which can lead to disease or symptoms.

White blood cells: All the cells of the immune system.

Window period: The time between HIV infection and seroconversion.

Bibliography

This bibliography was created to help the reader who is seeking additional information on the topics covered in the text. In many cases, the bibliography only serves as a starting point, and will steer you to articles or books that contain bibliographies of their own for additional information.

Most of the research cited is dated within the last two years to reflect the latest scientific findings on HIV.

Chapter 1: Hiring a Physician

ACT UP, "US HealthCare: An International Scandal," *Critical Path AIDS Project,* vol. 2, no. 9–10 (December 1991): 16.

Bennett, Charles L., et al., "Intensity of In-Hospital Care for Persons with AIDS," *Journal of AIDS,* vol. 4, no. 9 (September 1991): 856.

Bennett, Charles L., et al., "Medical Care Costs of Intravenous Drug Users with AIDS in Brooklyn," *Journal of AIDS,* vol. 5, no. 1 (January 1992): 1.

Fowlkes, Earl D., Jr., "Reaching Out to the Disenfranchised Infected and Affected by HIV/AIDS," *The Body Positive,* vol. 4, no. 10 (November 1991): 23.

Lewis, Jim, and Michael Slocum, "You Are Not Alone," *The Body Positive,* vol. 5, no. 11 (December 1992): 2. This article has been published monthly since 1991.

NDRI, *AIDS and Substance Abuse: Counseling Issues* (New York: Narcotic & Drug Research Institute Training Manual, 1989).

Project Inform, "Doctor, Patient and HIV: Building a Cooperative Relationship," Project Inform Discussion Paper, no. 3 (April 1988).

PWA Coalition, "Paying for Your Insurance—or NOT!" *PWA Newsline,* issue 78 (July 1992): 28.

Siano, Nick, "The Fatalistic Attitude of the Medical Community," *PWA Newsline,* issue 67 (July 1991): 41.

Spindell, Gail, C.S.W., "HIV Support Groups," *The Body Positive,* vol. 4, no. 3 (March 1991): 21.

Trzebiatowski, Daniel, "Picking a Direction," *PWA Newsline,* issue 78 (July 1992): 19.

Zwickler, Phil, and David Wojnarowicz, "Fear of Disclosure," *The Body Positive,* vol. 3, no. 11 (December 1990): 11.

Chapter 2: HIV: An Overview

ACT UP, "A Capsule History of ACT UP," ACT UP/New York new member information packet, 1991.

Balachadron, R., et al., "HIV Isolates from Asymptomatic Homosexual Men and from AIDS Patients Have Distinct Biologic and Genetic Properties," *CDC AIDS Weekly* (February 11, 1991): 19.

Boon, Marcus, "NAC and Apoptosis," *PWA Newsline,* issue 81 (October 1992): 50.

Boon, Marcus, and Kate Hunter, "Pathogenesis," PWA Newsline, issue 70 (October 1991): 46.

Harvard-Amsterdam Conference, *Final Program and Oral Abstracts,* vol. 1 (Amsterdam: Eighth International AIDS Conference, 1992).

Harvard-Amsterdam Conference, *Poster Abstracts,* vol. 2 (Amsterdam: Eighth International AIDS Conference, 1992).

Harvard-Amsterdam Conference, *Published Abstracts and Indices,* vol. 3 (Amsterdam: Eighth International AIDS Conference, 1992).

Kaplan, Jonathan E., et al., "Ten-Year Follow-up of HIV-Infected Homosexual Men with Lymphadenopathy Syndrome: Evidence for Continuing Risk of Developing AIDS," *Journal of AIDS,* vol. 5, no. 6 (June 1992): 565.

Kraus, Jeffrey, "AIDS Without HIV: A Tremor, Not an Earthquake," *ARCS News* (Fall 1992): 6.

Lewis, Jim, "Understanding HIV," *The Body Positive,* vol. 4, no. 6 (June 1991): 10.

Miller, Christopher, et al., "AIDS and Mucosal Immunity," *Journal of AIDS,* vol. 4, no. 12 (December 1991): 1169.

Morgan, Andrew, "I Want Your Sex!!!" *PWA Newsline,* issue 65 (May 1991): 21.

NDRI, *Human Sexuality and Safer Sex* (New York: Narcotic & Drug Research Institute Training Manual, 1989).

New York City Department of Health, "AIDS Surveillance Update:

Second Quarter 1992" (NYC Office of AIDS Surveillance, July 31, 1992).

New York State Department of Health, *A Physician's Guide to AIDS: Issues in the Medical Office* (New York State Department of Health, March 1988).

PWA Coalition, "News/Analysis: Surveys on Gay/Bisexual Knowledge of AIDS-Related Information and Practices," *PWA Newsline*, issue 69 (September 1991): 7.

Samuel, Michael C., et al., "Changes in Sexual Practices Over 5 Years of Follow-Up Among Heterosexual Men in San Francisco," *Journal of AIDS*, vol. 4, no. 9 (September 1991): 896.

Shilts, Randy, *And the Band Played On* (New York: St. Martin's Press, 1987).

Chapter 3: The Immune System

Baker, Ronald A., Ph.D., "AIDS, Cytokines and Chronic Fatigue Syndrome," *BETA* (February 1992): 7.

Bartlett, John G., M.D., and Ann K. Finkbeiner, *The Guide to Living with HIV Infection* (Baltimore, Md.: The Johns Hopkins University Press, 1991).

Burnis, Allan, "Too Much Assumption Too Little Known," *The Body Positive*, vol. 4, no. 7 (July/August 1991): 17.

Caldwell, John, "Co-Factors at the VI International," *PI Perspective*, no. 9 (October 1990): 17.

Frank-Ruta, Garance, "Tobacco Smoking and HIV Disease," *Treatment Issues*, vol. 6, no. 11 (December 1992): 7.

Hosein, Sean, "The Thymus Gland and HIV," *The Body Positive*, vol. 3, no. 11 (December 1990): 8.

McKean, Aldyn, "Report from Amsterdam," *The Body Positive*, vol. 5, no. 10 (November 1992): 10.

NDRI, *AIDS: Overview* (New York: Narcotic & Drug Research Institute Training Manual, 1989).

Project Inform, "Immune Restoration: Conference Report," *PI Perspective*, no. 10 (April 1991): 17.

Project Inform, "Restoring the Immune System: Concepts and a Conference," *PI Perspective*, no. 9 (October 1990): 11.

The Science of AIDS: Readings from Scientific American (New York: W. H. Freeman, 1989).

Treatment Issues: Compilation Issue, November 1987–January 1991 (New York: Gay Men's Health Crisis, 1991).

Volberding, Paul, and Mark A. Jacobson, *AIDS Clinical Review 1992* (New York: Marcel Dekker, Inc., 1992).

Chapter 4: HIV Evolution and Symptoms: An Overview

ACT UP/Philadelphia, "HIV Standard of Care," *Critical Path AIDS Project,* vol. 3, no. 4 (April 1992): 1.

Baker, Ronald A., Ph.D., "Review of the Epidemiology of Kaposi's Sarcoma," *BETA* (November 1992): 23.

Britton, Darren, "Mycobacterium Avium Complex," *Treatment Issues,* vol. 5, no. 8 (November 1991): 1.

Cardinale, Marisa, "CRIA Studies Pentoxifylline," *CRIA Update* (Winter 1992): 2.

Clardy, Tonisa, "Tuberculosis: A Second Epidemic?" *PI Perspective,* no. 12 (April 1992): 4.

"Consideration in the Management of Some Signs and Symptoms, in Patients With Low T_4's," *The Body Positive,* vol. 4, no. 7 (July/August 1991): 29.

Dunne, Richard, and Carole Lemens, "Progressive Multifocal Leukoencephalopathy (PML)," *Treatment Issues,* vol. 4, no. 6 (August 30, 1990): 4.

Lynch, Catherine, "Proposed Definition of AIDS: A Better Fit for Women, Poor People, and Injection Drug Users," *Treatment Issues,* vol. 6, no. 11 (December 1992): 11.

Portolano, Frank X., "Opportunistic Infections and Current Treatment Options," AIDS Training Institute (New York City Department of Health, May 1991).

Project Inform, "New Definition of AIDS," *PI Perspective,* no. 11 (October 1991): 10.

Project Inform, "Preface: Guide to OI's," *PI Perspective,* no. 11 (October 1991): 11.

Read, Stanley E., et al., "Comparison of Three HIV Antigen Detection Kits in Sequential Sera from a Cohort of Homosexual Men," *Journal of AIDS,* vol. 4, no. 7 (July 1991): 717.

Shewey, Don, "Neuropathies in HIV Patients," *Treatment Issues,* vol. 5, no. 5 (June 20, 1991): 3.

Chapter 5: Monitoring Your Treatment

Armington, Kevin, "Surrogate Markers: Overview and Update," *Treatment Issues,* vol. 6, no. 1 (January 1992): 2.

Baker, Ronald A., Ph.D., "Advances in the Use of Polymerase Chain Reaction Technology," *BETA* (November 1992): 25.

Baker, Ronald A., Ph.D., "Low T-Helper Cell Counts Predictive of Survival," *BETA* (November 1992): 26.

Baker, Ronald A., Ph.D., "Research Notes," *BETA* (February 1991): 13.

Crowe, Suzanne M., "Predictive Value of CD4 Lymphocyte Numbers for the Development of Opportunistic Infections and Malignancies in HIV-Infected Persons," *Journal of AIDS*, vol. 4, no. 8 (August 1991): 770.

Dawson, Jeffrey D., and Stephen W. Lagakos, "Analyzing Laboratory Marker Changes in AIDS Clinical Trials," *Journal of AIDS*, vol. 4, no. 7 (July 1991): 667.

Hendrix, Craig W., et al., "HIV Antigen Variability in ARC/AIDS," *Journal of AIDS*, vol. 4, no. 9 (September 1991): 847.

James, John S., *AIDS Treatment News Compilation* (Berkeley, CA: Celestial Arts, 1989), issues 1–75.

Kramer, Alexander, et al., "Neopterin: A Predictive Marker of AIDS in HIV Infection," *Journal of AIDS*, vol. 2, no. 3 (1989): 291.

Longini, Ira M., et al., "The Dynamics of CD4+ T-Lymphocyte Decline in HIV-Infected Individuals," *Journal of AIDS*, vol. 4, no. 11 (November 1991): 1141.

Martin, David H., "Sequential Measurement of B2-Microglobulin Levels, P24 Antigen Levels, and Antibody Titers Following Transplantation of an HIV-Infected Kidney Allograft," *Journal of AIDS*, vol. 4, no. 11 (November 1991): 1118.

Masur, Henry, M.D., et al., "CD4 Counts as Predictors of Opportunistic Pneumonias in HIV Infection," *Annals of Internal Medicine*, vol. 111, no. 3 (August 1, 1989): 223.

McCutchan, Francine E., et al., "Genetic Comparison of HIV-1 Isolates by Polymerase Chain Reaction," *Journal of AIDS*, vol. 4, no. 12 (December 1991): 1241.

Phillips, Andrew N., "The Cumulative Risk of AIDS as the CD4 Lymphocyte Count Declines," *Journal of AIDS*, vol. 5, no. 2 (February 1992): 148.

Powell, Matt, "Common Laboratory Tests," *PWA Newsline*, issue 69 (September 1991): 31.

Project Inform, "Supplement on Testing," Project Inform Discussion Paper (October 11, 1988).

Siano, Nick, "How to Monitor the Effectiveness of Your Treatment Options," *PWA Newsline*, issue 74 (March 1992): 40.

Taylor, Jeremy, M.D., et al., "CD4 Percentage, CD4 Number and CD4: CD8 Ratio in HIV Infection: Which to Choose and How to Use," *Journal of AIDS*, vol. 2, no. 2 (1989): 114.

Chapter 6: The Range of Treatment Options

Armington, Kevin, "New Treatments: Evaluation and Access," *Treatment Issues*, vol. 5, no. 3 (March 28, 1991): 6.

Glassberg, David, "Clinical Trials: Evaluating, Choosing, Entering," *PI Perspective*, no. 7 (November 1989): 12.

Lasagna, Louis, M.D., et al., "A Call to Reform Drug Testing," *BETA* (November 1990): 16.

Project Inform, "Expedited Drug Approval—What It Is and Why It Matters," *PI Perspective,* no. 11 (October 1991).

Project Inform, "FDA: ddI, ddC; NDA—ASAP, RSVP!" *PI Perspective,* no. 9 (October 1990).

Project Inform, "HIV Treatment Strategy," Project Inform Discussion Paper, no. 1 (January 12, 1989).

Volberding, Paul A., M.D., "Management of Early HIV Disease," *BETA* (April 1992): 1.

Chapter 7: Acupuncture, Chiropractic, Chinese Medicine, and Homeopathy

Badgley, Laurence E., *Healing AIDS Naturally* (Foster City, CA: Human Energy Press: 1987).

Burroughs, Carola, "Mechanisms of Holistic Healing," *PWA Newsline,* issue 39 (December 1988): 33.

Franchino, Charles, D.C., "Chiropractic and HIV," *PWA Newsline,* issue 56 (June 1990): 30.

Horral, Craig, "Holistics," *PI Perspective,* no. 9 (October 1990): 17.

Institute for Traditional Medicine, "Chinese Herbal Therapies for HIV," *The Body Positive,* vol. 3, no. 10 (November 1990): 13.

Lederer, Bob, "A Clove a Day: Garlic, AIDS and Politics," *Outweek* (January 16, 1991).

Scheru, Prisicilla, R.N., "Acupuncture," *Treatment Issues,* vol. 5, no. 4 (June 1991): 4.

The Science of AIDS: Readings from Scientific American (New York: W. H. Freeman and Company, 1989).

Slocum, Michael, "Alternative & Holistic Therapies," *The Body Positive,* vol. 4, no. 6 (June 1991): 16.

Zhang, Qingcai, M.D., and Hong-yen Hsu, Ph.D., *AIDS and Chinese Medicine* (Berkeley, Calif.: Oriental Healing Arts Institute, 1990).

Chapter 8: Natural Interventions

ACT UP/NY, "Vitamin B_{12} and Its Importance to People Who Are HIV-Positive," ACT UP/New York Treatment Alternatives Packet (September 1991).

ACT UP/NY, "Vitamin C," ACT UP/New York Treatment Alternatives Packet (September 1991).

ACT UP/NY, "Hypericin," ACT UP/New York Treatment Alternatives Packet (September 1991).

ACT UP/NY, "Glycyrrhizin," ACT UP/New York Treatment Alternatives Packet (July 1991).

Altman, Lawrence K., "Chemicals Stop Growth of AIDS Virus in Test," *New York Times,* Washington Talk (August 16, 1989).

Baker, Ronald A., Ph.D., "Vitamin B_{12} in HIV Infection," *BETA* (November 1990): 24.

Baum, Marianna K., et al., "Association of Vitamin B Status with Parameters of Immune Function in Early HIV-1 Infection," *Journal of AIDS,* vol. 4, no. 11 (November 1991): 1122.

Bihari, Bernard, M.D., "Hypericin for the Treatment of HIV Disease: An Update," *BETA* (May 1992): 33.

"Biomedicine: Blue-Green Algae Kill HIV in Culture," *Science News* (August 26, 1989).

"Blue-Green Algae May Provide Medical Breakthroughs," *Fairborn Daily Herald* (May 3, 1988).

Blume, Anna, "Hypericin Trial in New York: At Last!" *Treatment Issues,* vol. 5, no. 9 (December 1991): 3.

Broder, Samuel, M.D., "NAC," *The Body Positive,* vol. 2, no. 8 (November 1989): 18.

Forefront, "Alternative Treatments for CMV," *PWA Newsline,* issue 82 (November 1992): 38.

Franulovich, Tim, "Glutothione Levels Raised with NAC," *The Body Positive,* vol. 4, no. 5 (May 1991): 14.

Garrity, Clelia P., "Vitamin C Makes a Comeback," *ARCS News* (January 1991): 2.

Goldberg, Billi, "Explanation: DNCB and the Immune System," *Critical Path AIDS Project,* vol. 3, nos. 2–3 (February/March 1992): 7.

Graham, Neil M. H., et al., "Relationship of Serum Copper and Zinc Levels to HIV-1 Seropositivity and Progression to AIDS," *Journal of AIDS,* vol. 4, no. 10 (October 1991): 976.

Greenberg, Jon M., "Vitamin B_{12}—Breakfast of Champions," *Outweek* (June 12, 1991): 28–29.

Hariman, et al., "Cobalamin Deficiency in HIV Patients," *American Society of Psychiatric Oncology/AIDS,* vol. 3, no. 2 (September 1991).

Hosein, Sein, "Vitamin C Found to Inhibit HIV Replication," *The Body Positive,* vol. 4, no. 5 (May 1991): 15.

James, John S., "Hypericin: Antiviral from St. John's Wort," *AIDS Treatment News International Edition* (July 1992).

James, John S., "Hypericin: Common Herb Shows Antiretroviral Activity," *AIDS Treatment News,* vol. 63 (August 1988).

James, John S., "Hypericin/St. John's Wort," *AIDS Treatment News,* vol. 73 (January 1989).

James, John S., "Hypericin Update," *AIDS Treatment News,* vol. 77 (April 1989).

Kuromuja, Kujoski, "The Nontoxic Path: Vitamins, Dietary Supplements, Adjunctive Therapies," *Critical Path AIDS Project*, vol. 3, nos. 2–3 (February/March 1992): 1.

Lands, Lark, Ph.D., "Blue-Green Algae," Therapeutic Basics for People Living with HIV/Carl Vogel Foundation (1989).

Lands, Lark, Ph.D., "Therapeutic Basics for People Living with HIV," *The Body Positive*, vol. 4, no. 7 (July/August 1991): 11.

Link, Derek, "NIC, NAC, Paddy Whack . . . ," *Notes from the Underground*, issue 16 (July/August 1992): 1.

"Scientists Say Algae Substance 'Strikingly Active' Against AIDS," *The Daily Progress*, National News Briefs (August 16, 1989).

Smith, Denny, "Zinc and B Vitamins in HIV: Overview and Interview," *AIDS Treatment News*, issue 134 (September 6, 1991): 5.

"Sulfolipids," *AIDS Therapies* (New York: Charles Henderson, 1991).

Chapter 9: Immune Modulators

Baker, Ronald A., Ph.D., "Immuthiol (DTC): Antiviral or Immunomodulator?" *BETA* (February 1991): 15.

Baker, Ronald A., Ph.D., "I.V. Gamma Globulin," *BETA* (November 1990): 24.

Bihari, Bernard, M.D., "Ambulatory Management of HIV Related Immune Suppression and AIDS," *The Body Positive*, vol. 4, no. 7 (July/August 1991): 13.

Bihari, Bernard, M.D., "Management of HIV Disease: One Physician's Approach," *BETA* (November 1991): 10.

Brust, Douglas G., Ph.D., "Cimetidine," *Treatment Issues*, vol. 6, no. 1 (January 1992): 8.

Dennis, Karen, "Naltrexone," *Treatment Issues*, vol. 4, no. 1 (January 29, 1990): 1.

Franke-Ruta, Garance, "L'Immuthiol: Le Fin?" *Notes from the Underground*, issue 12 (November/December 1991): 8.

Franke-Ruta, Garance, "L'Immuthiol: Pas Encore!" *Notes from the Underground*, issue 11 (September/October 1991).

Franke-Ruta, Garance, et al., "RUN DTC," *Notes from the Underground*, issue 4 (July 1990): 6.

Franke-Ruta, Garance, "Undergrowth: Levamisole," *Notes from the Underground*, issue 9 (May 1991).

James, John S., "Gamma Globulin to Prevent Infections?" *AIDS Treatment News*, issue 152 (June 5, 1992): 1.

Project Inform, Naltrexone (Trexan), Project Inform Fact Sheet.

Chapter 10: Antiviral Options

ACT UP/NY, "Peptide T Availability, Packaging, and Dosing Information," ACT UP/New York Treatment Alternatives Packet (September 1991).

AmFAR, *AIDS/HIV Treatment Directory,* vol. 6, no. 1 (New York: American Foundation for AIDS Research, September 30, 1992).

Armington, Kevin, "Combination Antiviral Therapy," *Treatment Issues,* vol. 4, no. 5 (July 30, 1990): 2.

Armington, Kevin, "News from Florence: Combination Antiviral Therapy," *Treatment Issues,* vol. 5, no. 6 (August 30, 1991): 1.

Baker, Ronald A., Ph.D., "Combination Therapy: A New Era in HIV Therapeutics," *BETA* (February 1991): 3.

Baker, Ronald A., Ph.D., "FDA Antiviral Advisory Committee Recommendations on ddC and ddI," *BETA* (May 1992): 31.

Baker, Ronald A., Ph.D., "FDA Approval of ddI (VIDEX)," *BETA* (November 1991): 28.

Baker, Ronald A., Ph.D., "Research Notes," *BETA* (November 1990): 19.

Beswick, Terry, "Aggressive Early Intervention—An Antiviral Approach," *PI Perspective,* no. 11 (October 1991): 10.

Blume, Anna, "Peptide T Available in New York," *Treatment Issues,* vol. 5, no. 8 (November 1991): 6.

Blume, Anna, "Update on Peptide T," *The Body Positive,* vol. 4, no. 5 (May 1991): 16.

Child, Stephen, et al., "Canadian Multicenter Azidothymedine Trial: AZT Pharmacokinetics," *Journal of AIDS,* vol. 4, no. 9 (September 1991): 865.

Fitzpatrick, Brian, and Derek Link, "Day of the HIVID," *Notes from the Underground,* issue 16 (July/August 1992): 6.

Franke-Ruta, Garance, et al., "Compound Q: Clinical Experience," *Notes from the Underground,* issue 9 (May 1991): 4.

Franke-Ruta, Garance, et al., "Quid Pro Q," *Notes from the Underground,* issue 8 (March 1991).

Franke-Ruta, Garance, "To a Peptide T . . . ," *Notes from the Underground,* issue 10 (July/August 1991): 5.

"In Brief: Lower-Dose AZT!," *Treatment Issues,* vol. 4, no. 7 (October 12, 1990): 7.

"In Brief: Pentoxifylline to Be Tested," *Treatment Issues,* vol. 5, no. 4 (May 15, 1991): 11.

James, John S., "ddC Approved for AZT Combinations," *AIDS Treatment News,* issue 154 (July 3, 1992): 1.

James, John S., "ddC Background," *AIDS Treatment News,* issue 145 (February 21, 1992): 3.

James, John S., "Pentoxifylline: AmFAR Supports CRIA Trial in New York," *AIDS Treatment News*, issue 145 (February 21, 1992): 8.

Kawadler, Wayne, "Peptide T Access Blocked," *Treatment Issues*, vol. 5, no. 1 (January 19, 1990): 1.

Little, Marjorie, "ddI—dideoxyinosine—(Videx)," Project Inform Fact Sheet (June 14, 1990).

Luder, Elizabeth, Ph.D., and Jamie Rodriquiz, "Compound Q Update," *Treatment Issues*, vol. 3, no. 6 (October 30, 1989): 9.

"Peptide T," *Treatment Issues*, vol. 3, no. 1, (February 6, 1989): 2.

Project Inform, "AZT—Retrovir," Project Inform Fact Sheet (March 27, 1990).

Project Inform, "Clinical Update," *PI Perspective*, no. 8 (May 1990).

Project Inform, "Combination Therapy: Why, How and When," *PI Perspective*, no. 10 (April 1991): 3.

Project Inform, "Compound Q—The Real Story," *PI Perspective*, no. 7 (November 1989).

Project Inform, "ddI Approval," *PI Perspective*, no. 11 (October 1991).

Project Inform, "The Clinical Trials of Compound Q: A Brief Synopsis," *PI Perspective*, no. 9 (October 1990): 14.

PWA Coalition, "Demand for Expanded Access to Peptide T," *PWA Newsline*, issue 68 (August 1991): 42.

PWA Health Group, "Peptide T," PWA Health Group Information Sheet (November 7, 1991).

Torres, Gabriel, M.D., "Antiviral Options: AZT, ddI, or ddC," *Treatment Issues*, vol. 5, no. 2 (February 25, 1991): 1.

Torres, Gabriel, M.D., "AZT/ddI Highlights from European AIDS Conference," *Treatment Issues*, vol. 6, no. 5 (May/June 1992): 1.

Torres, Gabriel, M.D., "AZT Resistance," *Treatment Issues*, vol. 4, no. 6 (August 30, 1990): 3.

Torres, Gabriel, M.D., "ddC Update," *Treatment Issues*, vol. 5, no. 5 (June 20, 1991): 1.

Torres, Gabriel, M.D., "ddI: Long-Term Effect," *Treatment Issues*, vol. 4, no. 7 (October 12, 1990): 1.

Torres, Gabriel, M.D., "VIII International Conference on AIDS: Antiretroviral Update," *Treatment Issues*, vol. 6, no. 8 (September 1992): 1.

Torres, Gabriel, M.D., "Life After FDA Approval: ddI Update," *Treatment Issues*, vol. 5, no. 9 (December 1991).

Wellcome PLC, "Genetic Basis for Resistance to Zidovudine," *CDC AIDS Weekly* (January 15, 1990): 5.

Chapter 11: Special Concerns of Women

Auer, Lisa, "Developing a Clinical Research Agenda for Women," *PI Perspective*, no. 9 (October 1990).

Auer, Lisa, "Pap Testing and Cervical Disease: Implications for Women with HIV," *PI Perspective,* no. 12 (April 1992): 6.

Caschetta, Mary Beth, "A Review of Reports on Women and HIV," *Treatment Issues,* vol. 6, no. 10 (November 1992): 2.

Caschetta, Mary Beth, "Clinical Manifestations of HIV Infection in Women," *Treatment Issues,* vol. 5, no. 1 (January 10, 1990): 3.

Deneberg, Risa, F.N.P., "Women and HIV-Related Conditions," *The Body Positive,* vol. 4, no. 6 (June 1991): 12.

Deneberg, Risa, F.N.P., "Women, Immunity, and Sex Hormones," *Treatment Issues,* special edition, vol. 6, no. 7 (Summer/Fall 1992): 6.

Deneberg, Risa, F.N.P., "Pregnancy and HIV," vol. 5, no. 6 (August 30, 1991).

Franke-Ruta, Garance, "HPV and Cervical Cancer," *Treatment Issues,* special edition, vol. 6, no. 7 (Summer/Fall 1992): 22.

Franke-Ruta, Garance, and Mary Beth Caschetta, "Pelvic Inflammatory Disease," *Treatment Issues,* special edition, vol. 6, no. 7 (Summer/Fall 1992): 19.

Hayes, Bill, "Women and HIV Disease," *BETA* (February 1992): 1.

Kelly, Patricia, F.N.P., "Fertility, Menstruation, and Birth Control in HIV," *Treatment Issues,* special edition vol. 6, no. 7 (Summer/Fall 1992): 10.

Kraus, Jeffrey, "HIV Infection and Women: Part 1," *ARCS News* (May 1992): 3.

Mitchell, Janet L., M.D., M.P.H., "Syphilis Treatment in HIV-Infected Women," *Treatment Issues,* special edition, vol. 6, no. 7 (Summer/Fall 1992): 17.

Nuckols, Teryl, "Human Papillomavirus Infection in Women with HIV," *BETA* (November 1992): 8.

Pearl, Monica, "Women at the VIII International Conference on AIDS: A Brief Overview," *The Body Positive,* vol. 5, no. 10 (November 1992): 13.

Wilson, Scott, and Brenda Lein, "HIV Disease in Women," *Treatment Issues,* special edition, vol. 6, no. 7 (Summer/Fall 1992): 1.

Chapter 13: OI Treatments

Agins, Bruce D., et al., "Effect of Combined Therapy . . . for Mycobacterium Avium Infection in Patients with AIDS," *Journal of Infectious Diseases,* vol. 159, no. 4 (April 1989).

Baker, Ronald A., Ph.D., "Notes on Research and Care," *BETA* (April 1990): 15–22.

Baker, Ronald A., Ph.D., "Research Notes," *BETA* (November 1992): 20.

Berman, Bonnie, "Mexitine: A Promising New Drug to Treat Symptoms of Peripheral Neuropathy," *PWA Newsline*, issue 69 (September 1991): 33.

Bloom, Jeffrey, et al., "The Diagnosis of Cytomegalovirus Retinitis," *Annals of Internal Medicine* (December 15, 1988): 963.

Coodley, Gregg, et al., "HIV-Associated Wasting," *Journal of AIDS*, vol. 4, no. 8 (August 1991): 826.

Goethe, Katherine E., "Neuropsychological and Neurological Function of HIV in Asymptomatic Individual," *Arch Neurol*, vol. 46 (February 1989): 129.

Gonsalves, Gregg, "Cryptosporidiosis: Treatment Update," *Treatment Issues*, vol. 6, no. 3 (March 1992): 1.

"In Brief: Low-Dose Bactrim," *Treatment Issues*, vol. 5, no. 2 (February 25, 1991): 11.

James, John S., "Foscarnet Study Finds Increased Survival," *AIDS Treatment News*, issue 138 (November 1, 1991): 1.

Kraus, Jeffrey, "HIV Infection and Multidrug Resistant TB (MDR-TB)," *ARCS News* (January 1992): 3.

Lemens, Carole, "PML Treatment Update," *Treatment Issues*, vol. 6, no. 3 (March 1992): 5.

Lugliani, Greg, "CMV Treatment Overview," *Treatment Issues*, vol. 6, no. 4 (April 1992): 7.

Loun, Laine, et al., "Cytomegalovirus and Candida Esophagitis in Patients with AIDS," *Journal of AIDS*, vol. 5, no. 6 (June 1992): 605.

Neger, Robert, M.D., "The Eye and HIV Infection," *BETA* (November 1990): 1.

Piette, John, et al., "Patterns of Secondary Prophylaxis with Aerosol Pentamidine Among Persons with AIDS," *Journal of AIDS*, vol. 4, no. 8 (August 1991): 826.

Project Inform, "A Note to Dr. Gallo on KS: Do the Right Thing!" *PI Perspective*, no. 8 (May 1990).

Project Inform, "Clinical Update," *PI Perspective*, no. 9 (October 1990): 9.

Project Inform, "CMV Retinitis," *PI Perspective*, no. 8 (May 1990): 17.

Project Inform, "Gallo Responds on KS," *PI Perspective*, no. 9 (October 1990): 5.

Project Inform, "Project Inform Guide to Management of Opportunistic Infections," *PI Perspective*, no. 8 (May 1990): 12.

Raviglione, Mario C., et al., "Infections Associated with Hickman Catheters in Patients with AIDS," *American Journal of Medicine*, vol. 86 (June 1989): 780.

Smith, Denny, "Azithromycin and Clarithromycin Approved," *AIDS Treatment News*, issue 139 (November 22, 1991): 1.

Torres, Gabriel, M.D., "Desensitization to Sulfa Drugs," *Treatment Issues*, vol. 6, no. 10 (November 1992): 6.

Torres, Gabriel, M.D., "Toxoplasmosis: New Treatment Advances," *Treatment Issues,* vol. 5, no. 3 (March 28, 1991): 1.

Waites, Dr. Larry, "Coping with MAI," *PI Perspective,* no. 8 (May 1990): 12.

Walmsley, Sharon, et al., "The Possible Role of Corticosteroid Function of HIV in Asymptomatic Individual," *Arch Neurol,* vol. 46 (February 1989): 129.

Chapter 14: Preventive Therapy

Baker, Ronald A., Ph.D., "Intravenous Ganciclovir to Prevent CMV Disease," *BETA* (February 1992): 23.

Bevilacqua, Francesca, "Acyclovir Resistance/Susceptibility in Herpes Simplex Virus Type 2 Sequential Isolates from an AIDS Patient," *Journal of AIDS,* vol. 4, no. 10 (October 1991): 967.

Cox, Spencer, "High-Dose Acyclovir Controversy," *Treatment Issues,* vol. 6, no. 2 (February 1992): 1.

Franke-Ruta, Garance, "Clarithromycin Resistance Found," *Notes from the Underground,* issue 13 (January/February 1992): 8.

Franke-Ruta, Garance, "Guerillamycin!" *Notes from the Underground,* issue 5 (September 1990): 4.

Link, Derek, "Mother, MAI I?" *Notes from the Underground,* issue 16 (July/August 1992): 8.

Nott, Victoria, "An Ounce of Prevention: Antifungal Prophylaxis," *Treatment Issues,* vol. 5, no. 2 (February 25, 1991): 3.

Pierce, Phillip, "O.I. Prophylaxis Overview," *Treatment Issues,* vol. 6, no. 4 (April 1992): 1.

Project Inform, "Acyclovir," Project Inform Fact Sheet (June 12, 1990).

Project Inform, "PCP Prophylaxis," Project Inform Fact Sheet (September 27, 1988).

Project Inform "Preventing OIs: A Key to Survival," *PI Perspective,* no. 10 (April 1991): 7.

Torres, Gabriel, M.D., "An Ounce of Prevention: Update on Prophylaxis for Fungal Infection," *Treatment Issues,* vol. 5, no. 7 (October 1991): 4.

Chapter 15: Nutrition and HIV

Bruens, Kurt, "Total Parenteral Nutrition," *PI Perspective,* no. 11 (October 1991): 14.

"Eat Well: Food Remedies to Common Problems for People with HIV/AIDS," volunteer newsletter, *The Body Positive,* vol. 3, no. 10 (November 1990): 21.

Franke-Ruta, Garance, "Marinol," *Notes from the Underground,* issue 13 (January/February 1992): 4.

Goeke, Mary, and Robin Goldberg, "Early Nutritional Intervention," *The Body Positive,* vol. 4, no. 3 (March 1991): 27.

James, John S., "Nutrition and AIDS: Some Information Sources," *AIDS Treatment News,* issue 134 (September 6, 1991): 1.

"Marijuana Therapy in HIV," *Treatment Issues,* vol. 5, no. 5 (June 20, 1991): 7.

Pierce, Richard, and Patrick Donnelly, "Diet, Cholesterol, and HIV: A Crash Course," *The Body Positive,* vol. 5, no. 10 (November 1992): 18.

Pierce, Richard, and Patrick Donnelly, "Whole Foods, HIV, and Digestive Problems," *The Body Positive,* vol. 5, no. 7 (July/August 1992): 16.

Torres, Gabriel, M.D., "Megace to Stimulate Appetite," *Treatment Issues,* vol. 5, no. 9 (December 1991): 8.

Veston, Diane L., "Nutrition, Vitamins, and Immunity," *ARCS News* (June 1991): 4.

Chapter 16: Infection Control

Lubell, Arthur, "Pet Care: Special Concerns for People with HIV Infection," *Treatment Issues,* vol. 5, no. 2 (February 25, 1991): 7.

NDRI, *AIDS: Medical Education for Health Care Providers* (New York: Narcotic & Drug Research Institute Training Manual, 1989).

Chapter 17: The Mind–Body Connection: Psychoneuroimmunology

Callen, Michael, *Surviving AIDS* (New York: HarperCollins, 1990).

Cousins, Norman, *Head First* (New York: E. P. Dutton, 1988).

Hay, Louise L., *AIDS: Creating a Positive Approach* (Carson, Calif.: Hay House, 1988).

Hay, Louise L., *You Can Heal Your Life* (Carson, Calif.: Hay House, 1987).

Lewis, Jim, "HIV/AIDS, A Blessing?" *The Body Positive,* vol. 5, no. 10 (November 1992): 5.

Nichols, Michael, "Disease, Denial and Death," *The Body Positive,* vol. 5, no. 10 (November 1992): 25.

Rabkin, Judith G., and Robert H. Remien, "Maintaining Hope: A Research Study," *The Body Positive,* vol. 3, no. 11 (December 1990): 20.

Siegel, Bernie S., M.D., *Love, Medicine, and Miracles* (New York: HarperCollins, 1990).

Slocum, Michael, "Stress," *The Body Positive,* vol. 3, no. 10 (November 1990): 17.

Williamson, Marianne, *A Return to Love* (New York: HarperCollins, 1992).

Chapter 18: On the Horizon

AmFAR, *New York State Directory of AIDS/HIV Clinical Trials,* vol. 2, no. 1 (New York: American Foundation for AIDS Research, Winter/Spring 1992).

Armington, Kevin, "Passive Immunotherapy Update," *Treatment Issues,* vol. 4, no. 4 (June 15, 1990): 1.

Baker, Ronald A., Ph.D., "SP-PG: A Promising Anti-KS Drug," *BETA* (May 1992): 25.

Franke-Ruta, Garance, "A New Tide in Antiviral Research," *Treatment Issues,* vol. 5, no. 4 (May 15, 1991): 1.

Hayes, Bill, "Vaccines for HIV," *BETA* (February 1991): 9.

James, John S., "1992: Treatments to Watch," *AIDS Treatment News,* issue 141 (December 20, 1991): 1.

James, John S., "Tat Inhibitor Update," *AIDS Treatment News,* issue 142 (January 3, 1992): 1.

James, John S., "Passive Hyperimmune Therapy (Passive Immunotherapy): New Data Released, California Approval Possible," *AIDS Treatment News,* issue 148 (April 3, 1992): 1.

James, John S., "Tat Drug Development: Current Status," *AIDS Treatment News,* issue 153 (June 19, 1992): 1.

Owens, Karl, "The Status of Tat," *Treatment Issues,* vol. 6, no. 3 (March 1992): 8.

Project Inform, "Clinical Update," *PI Perspective,* no. 12 (April 1992): 14.

Ravitch, Michael, "D4T Overview," *Treatment Issues,* vol. 6, no. 10 (November 1992): 1.

Torres, Gabriel, M.D., "566c80: New Weapon Against PCP and Toxoplasmosis," *Treatment Issues,* vol. 6, no. 1 (January 1992): 1.

Torres, Gabriel, M.D., "Update on Vaccine Development," *Treatment Issues,* vol. 5, no. 6 (August 30, 1991): 3.

Torres, Gabriel, M.D., "Vaccine Developments," *Treatment Issues,* vol. 6, no. 7 (September 1992): 7.

Chapter 19: Keeping Current

Malinowsky, Robert H., and Gerald J. Perry, *AIDS: Information Sourcebook,* third edition, 1991–92 (Phoenix, Ariz.: Oryx Press, 1991).

New York City Department of Health, "AIDS Forum Newsletter," New York City Division of AIDS Program Services (April/May 1991).

Project Inform, "Project Inform: A History," Project Inform Fact Sheet (1990).

Thomas, Laura, and Denny Smith, "Resource List, January 1992," *AIDS Treatment News*, issue 143 (January 1992): 6.

Index

About the Authors

Nick Siano, a certified HIV counselor, writes and lectures nationally on HIV treatments with an emphasis on the latest developments in alternative and mainstream HIV treatment options. He is regularly consulted by medical professionals in search of updated information on HIV treatment, and is currently the HIV specialist at Friends In Deed in New York City. Prior to that, he was the HIV specialist at HELP/Project Samaritan, the first residential drug-treatment program in the United States for symptomatic HIV+ people. He lives in Brooklyn, New York.

Suzanne Lipsett is a California-based writer, with a particular interest in health issues. Her latest titles include *Remember Me* (Mercury House, 1991), a novel, and *Surviving a Writer's Life* (forthcoming from Harper San Francisco), an essay collection on memory, imagination, and writing. She lives in Petaluma, California.